GOOD INTENTIONS OVERRULED:
A CRITIQUE OF EMPOWERMENT IN THE
ROUTINE ORGANIZATION OF MENTAL HEALTH SERVICES

Good Intentions OverRuled is about empowerment; so it is also about power. This book shows how power is exerted in the routine organizational processes that determine what can be done in everyday life, since modern societies are controlled by regulations, policies, professional practice, legislation, budgets, and other forms of organization.

Against the backdrop of an ideal vision of empowerment, this critique highlights both the *good intentions* of professionals and the organizational processes through which empowerment is *overruled*. Professionals who promote empowerment for those with little power, such as people with long-standing mental health problems, experience tension, a disjuncture between *enabling participation* in empowerment and engaging in *caregiving* processes that perpetuate dependence. Attempts to enable participation are undermined by processes of objectification, individualized accountability, hierarchical decision making, simulation-based education, risk management, and exclusion, which protect but also control people. The significance of this critique extends beyond mental health services because similar processes are used in the routine organization of power in education, employment insurance, transportation, and other sectors of society.

Good Intentions OverRuled sparks debate about empowerment by using a method called *institutional ethnography*, developed by the Canadian sociologist Dorothy Smith. Mental health day programs are explored from the standpoint of seven occupational therapists in Atlantic Canada. Described in this ethnography are the local, provincial, federal, and international processes used to organize power in Canada's mental health services. The aim is to inspire professional, lay, academic, and other persons (including those who use mental health services) to change the organization of power so that we promote rather than overrule empowerment.

ELIZABETH TOWNSEND

Good Intentions OverRuled: A Critique of Empowerment in the Routine Organization of Mental Health Services

UNIVERSITY OF TORONTO PRESS
Toronto Buffalo London

© University of Toronto Press Incorporated 1998
Toronto Buffalo London
Printed in Canada

ISBN 0-8020-0753-8 (cloth)
ISBN 0-8020-7802-8 (paper)

Printed on acid-free paper

Canadian Cataloguing in Publication Data

Townsend, Elizabeth A., 1945–
    Good intentions overruled : a critique of empowerment
in the routine organization of mental health services

    Includes bibliographical references and index.
    ISBN 0-8020-0753-8 (bound)   ISBN 0-8020-7802-8 (pbk.)

    1. Mental health services – Canada.   2. Social medicine –
United States.   I. Title.

RA790.7.C3T69 1997   362.1'042   C97-931316-3

University of Toronto Press acknowledges the financial assistance to its
publishing program of the Canada Council for the Arts and the Ontario
Arts Council.

This book has been published with the help of a grant from the Humanities and Social Sciences Federation of Canada, using funds provided by
the Social Sciences and Humanities Research Council of Canada.

Contents

Figures

Foreword

More years ago than I care to think about I did the field research for my doctoral thesis in a large state mental hospital in California. Those residential warehouses for the mentally ill have now largely disappeared and among the otherwise displaced people in our society, we meet, as homeless people on the street, some at least of those who would in the past have been the inhabitants of what were called then 'chronic' wards. It is true that the hospital provided food, shelter, and health care. At the same time it was a kind of institutionalized disaster. I remember when one of the other large state hospitals in California was closed and its 'inmates' had to be housed elsewhere. Some fifty were sent to the hospital I was working at. About twenty of the 'chronic' patients were shipped into the hospital without records. Their records had long been lost. They themselves had no speakable memory. Nameless, without speech, lacking agency, they were the products of the traditional practices of warehousing the 'mentally ill.'

At that time, the state mental hospital I was working at was a leader in programs returning people housed there to the community. In so doing they were up against the contradictions that Elizabeth Townsend locates in new forms. In the hospitals, on the ward, patients were in 'custody.' This was a formal status that assigned responsibility for their care and behaviour to the hospital and its staff, a responsibility full of ambiguities, sometimes even involving the exercise of force against the patient. For example, one who refused to go to meals would be first pressured and then, if she resisted, strong-armed into the dining room. The individual's function of agency was appropriated by the institution. Every act of will on the part of the patient either was an act of resistance or was undercut by its representation of an institutional 'will.' Patients occupied the curious status of inmates, those who are 'in' the organization: the objects of its work, but never participants.

Elizabeth Townsend's institutional ethnography explores the continuities of this dilemma some thirty-five years later and under very different conditions. Patients are no longer confined indefinitely. With the help of medications, hospitalizations can be limited and the patient returned to her or his life in the community. In the hospital setting of old, occupational therapists provided ways of making bearable the long, long hours of inertia. Under the new regime they play a new and much more significant role, at the intersection of the institutional order of psychiatry with the everyday realities of living and working in the community. It is the professional and, as Townsend makes clear, the wonderfully personal commitment of occupational therapists to work with patients toward patients' self-activity, competence, and ability to take responsibility for their own lives. They work against difficulties created by reductions in funding for their and related services, by aspects of the society and economy which make uphill work for those disadvantaged by being already 'excluded,' and, as Townsend's analysis demonstrates, by dimensions of the institutional order that they are part of and are responsible for 'enforcing.' They work also against damage already done to patients' self-esteem and confidence that is incidental to the mental disorder from which they suffer.

Striking as are the improvements of these new forms of psychiatric service over the old, the institutional regime that Townsend displays still confronts the same fundamental contradictions. Occupational therapists work at just that site where the contradictions I've described emerge as practical and professional issues. On the one hand, there is an institutional order that individuates patients, objectifies them as 'cases,' and reduces them to the passive, non-participatory role that patients play when they are institutionalized objects of psychiatric care, and on the other, the discourse of and commitment to empowerment that can only be actualized 'out there' in the 'community.' Here, I thought as I read, are inmates again. But they are no longer confined by the hospital's walls, barred windows, and locked doors. New approaches, and above all, new medications, make it possible to avoid 'institutionalization' for the majority of people who experience mental illness (unless we count the streets of the city where people who are mentally ill live in varying states of ruin as a new form of 'institutionalization'). The new institutional practices create the new inmates, those who live in the community or are in preparation to do so, but at the same time, in their role as patients, have had their capacities as agents appropriated by the institution. Others have taken responsibility for their treatment and care in ways that in the case of mental illness are not well defined or clearly demarcated. The contradiction is embedded in the practices and the objectives of occupational therapy and becomes part of the ordinary and everyday problems to be solved for each and every patient. They strive to make it possible for individuals who are mentally ill to live autonomously, and at the same time are caught up in the institutional appropriation of the patient's agency. They struggle with the intimacies of these contradictions in the very practices of their profession. As Townsend describes them, occupational therapists are ingenious in developing exercises for the patient through which they acquire bit by bit the competences they need to get around in the community and the confidence they need to use them. Often these are the practical skills of everyday life that most take for granted – getting around on public transportation or speaking on the telephone, for example. In their professional capacity, occupational therapists seek to direct 'patients' in the progressive acquisition of the skills they need in order to be able to function in the community without direction. But to direct is to deprive patients of precisely the experience of autonomy that the therapist is working to promote.

Psychiatry operates as a self-sealing system. Its focus individualized the 'patient,' disconnecting the problems, experiences, and outcomes of those who are mentally ill from the power relations necessarily embedded in its institutional regimes. Townsend is clear that the issues for patients are those of empowerment both within the institutional regime of psychiatry and in the community. The passivities of the former are in synergy with exclusions arising from the stigma of 'mental illness' and from the progressive effects of uneven participation in paid work. As we know, unemployment itself produces failures of self-esteem and confidence. It is the professional commitment of occupational therapy to help patients toward empowerment. But empowerment isn't a one-sided matter that patients can achieve by themselves. Empowerment is as much a condition of community and institution as of individuals. If people who are mentally ill have a hard time getting employment, this isn't just because of problems they may have, or of the stigma associated with being mentally ill. It is also an effect of the inequalities of work opportunities and services that are created in the society by how the economy of capitalism works and how government manages society for capital. Disempowerment is as much a product of social and economic conditions as of individual situations. There are political issues here and although the occupational therapists who were involved in Townsend's study are active in the community as advocates for the mentally ill, those designated as mentally ill themselves are not similarly empowered.

'Institutional ethnography' is a method of inquiry exploring the ways in which people's work participates in the ruling relations. 'Ruling relations' is a term that directs attention to social relations that enter into and organize the local settings of people's work so as to articulate them to orders of discourse and/or large-scale organization that govern multiple settings. 'Institutional ethnography' proposes to 'describe the ways ruling and management are actually done' (Campbell & Manicom, 1995, p. 13) as they appear and organize the local settings of people's work and experience. In developing her institutional ethnography of the work of occupational therapy, Townsend analyses the contradictions between the regime within which occupational therapists work for the practical empowerment of patients, and the actual conditions of the empowerment of those they work with. She recognizes the real dilemmas of their practice as arising not exclusively from within the realm of psychiatry but as intersecting with the political and economic situations of the communities in which they are working. Their clients' empowerment runs up against barriers that implicate relations of power other than those of psychiatry. Here issues go beyond those ordinarily recognized as professional. They are issues for citizens and as much therefore for those designated as mentally ill as for those who work toward helping them bridge the gap between the incapacitations of psychiatric institutions and the ideal of the individual empowered as her or his own agent. Townsend's investigation and analysis conclude with a bold political call for achieving the real conditions of empowerment for those who are designated mentally ill.

DOROTHY E. SMITH

Preface

A preface is an opportunity to speak directly to readers. In this case, I have two questions.

Who are you?

Are some of you sociologists? Maybe, like me, you find institutional ethnographies intriguing because they tell us how the world works – and thus how it might be changed to make life fairer for us all.

Maybe some of you are adult educators who recognize that empowerment is a process of learning to live differently than we now do. You will see that the book explores possibilities and constraints for *empowerment education*. Although the examples used are concerned with educating adults in mental health services, the analysis applies to adult education in schools as well as to the many sites that are not labelled 'education' or 'school' but where adults learn about power and powerlessness.

My hope is that some of you are managers. You may be attracted to this text because of your specific concern with the management of mental health services. Hopefully, you will think about (and encourage your friends who are managers in other institutions to think about) how management practices determine possibilities for empowerment. Large-scale, modern organizations need to be managed. Do we have the collective understanding and will to introduce radically different ways of managing so that hierarchies are turned on their side to make empowerment a reality?

What about those of you who are professionals? Possibly your work is in mental health services. I believe that professionals are necessary and inevitable in modern society. They gather knowledge and experience that generally are applied with the best of intentions. Yet professional work is full of traps and breeds elitist assumptions that professionals are the *only* people who know what is best.

If you are not a professional, are you what we call these days a *consumer*? Are you a mental health consumer, meaning that you have had difficulties that are attributed to a mental disorder or mental health problem? Consumers are increasingly active in examining institutions like mental health services. Your interest in this book is welcome since we need you to press for change in the way professional and management features of mental health services are organized.

I will end my speculation by asking if some of you are occupational therapists. Occupational therapy provides the *illustration*, the actual everyday practice, from which social organization is unravelled. The analysis in this book is not limited to occupational therapy; nevertheless, occupational therapy demonstrates both the potential and pitfalls for professionals who view empowerment as a foundation for healthy living.

Who Am I?

I am one of today's hybrids, working in what is currently called an interdisciplinary framework. My specialty for 30 years has been occupational therapy since graduating with a Diploma in Physical and Occupational Therapy (1967) and a Bachelor of Science (Occupational Therapy) (1979) from the University of Toronto. Almost 20 years ago, after working in Newfoundland, Alberta, and Ontario, I decided to augment my basic professional qualifications with graduate education. At the time, I was working in Prince Edward Island and was thrilled to discover that Saint Francis Xavier University in Antigonish, Nova Scotia, only a ferry ride from P.E.I., offered a Masters in Adult Education degree, which I could complete through distance learning.

It became immediately clear to me that there are great parallels between adult education and occupational therapy. The principles, processes, and aims of adult education are the foundations of occupational therapy approaches with adults. Rather than talking directly about education, however, occupational therapists describe our work as *enabling occupation*, that is, helping people to participate in choosing and engaging in meaningful and useful occupations in their environment. As adult educators, our intention is to enable people to prevent, live with, or overcome personal and social barriers related to mental or physical disability, aging, or social disadvantage. The term *occupation* is used broadly in its pre-industrial sense, referring to *all* the occupations in daily life. Occupation, like work, is more than a paid job, in that we occupy our time and place in this world in many occupations – looking after ourselves, caring for others, creating communities, establishing homes and families, having fun, and generating income.

In 1982, I moved to Halifax to help found the School of Occupational Therapy at Dalhousie University, where, in July 1997, I became the Director. By 1994, I had completed doctoral work in the sociological foundations of adult education by analysing the social organization of occupational therapy's mental health work. Since then, my work has continued to connect occupational therapy, adult education, and sociology, using participatory methods of education and research to explore how power works in the everyday occupations of mental health services and other sectors.

I am indebted to many people who contributed at various stages of this book. The study reported here would not have taken place without the courageous participation of seven occupational therapists and the managers who gave me access to mental health services. I was greatly aided in the analysis by the perceptive critique of Ann Manicom, my doctoral thesis supervisor and a former student of Dorothy Smith, who formulated the theory and method of institutional ethnography used here. Joseph Murphy and Michael Welton, both committee members for my thesis, provided invaluable insights as the analysis developed. Barbara O'Shea and all my colleagues and friends at the School of Occupational Therapy have shared my excitement as the thesis and now the book emerged. Linda Pentz, Yvonne Ling, and Nadine Knight provided helpful office and library assistance. Virgil Duff, Executive Editor at the University of Toronto Press, made the book possible through his enthusiasm and support. Thanks also to Barbara Porter at the University of Toronto Press and to James Leahy, who edited the book.

The last word of thanks goes to friends and family. Friends, particularly in Prince Edward Island, have provided long-term support. My parents, Betty and Fred Townsend, actually taught me fundamentals of empowerment by insisting that I expect to be treated and to treat others with respect and fairness. My mother's 'will of iron' (dubbed by my father) and my father's courage to turn impractical ideas into reality have left a lasting mark. My husband Harold Robertson and step-children Jean and Kelvin provide me with unending encouragement.

Funding for the doctoral work that forms the basis for this book was gratefully received from:

Canadian Occupational Therapy Foundation
   Thelma Cardwell Award
   Graduate Scholarship

Dalhousie University
   Special Killam Scholarship

National Health Research and Development Program
   Doctoral Fellowship

ELIZABETH (LIZ) TOWNSEND
Halifax, Nova Scotia
January 1997

GOOD INTENTIONS OVERRULED

1

Exploring Empowerment

Enabling Participation versus Caregiving

He doesn't know how to get people involved. He's essentially a caregiver.
(Jill)

Jill[1] points to two fundamentally different ways of helping. One way involves people by enabling participation. Rather than give care to dependent recipients, we can facilitate, guide, coach, encourage, or support people to participate in helping themselves. Processes that enable participation can be described by adapting an old proverb: *You can care for people for a day. But, if you educate people to become involved, you have helped them to care for themselves and others for a lifetime.* Participation engages people as activists in shaping their own lives. In contrast to the one-way dependence that underlies caregiving, participation is enabled in two-way, interdependent processes that generate empowerment for us all.

In contrast, caregiving needs an object of care. We all need care in infancy, in crises, or in situations of specialized need. There are times when we need to be nurtured and protected if we are to grow or heal. However, health care, social welfare, and many volunteer agencies make us caregivers, caring for people in a one-way process of helping. Caregiving can be reciprocated, but reciprocity and mutual helping are not inherent in caregiving. Those who are objects of care can remain passive, dependent recipients of that care.

To enable participation is to work *with* people, to unleash human resources in the interests of empowerment; to be a caregiver is to offer charity *to* or *for* people who remain dependent. Some may say that the differences between these two approaches are minor, or too theoretical to worry about; however, for education, human service, health, and other professionals who want to help others, the differences form an underlying tension that pervades everyday practice. At its heart, this book shows how the tension between enabling participation and caregiving is routinely organized in mental health services.

Studying Empowerment from Points of Tension

I discovered the tension between enabling participation and caregiving while studying empowerment in the work of occupational therapists who practise in mental health services. The study, which forms the basis of this book, is summarized in the last section of this chapter. However, let us first hear how this tension was experienced by the seven occupational therapists whose practice provided my entry point for understanding how mental health services are organized in Canada's Atlantic Region, in the context of this country's national health system.

Jill highlighted the tension in her statement that opens this chapter. Drawing on comments from each of the seven occupational therapists in the study, we can hear key dimensions and variations in the way this tension is experienced. As Jill talks more about her work, she does not mention an underlying, socially organized tension. Rather, she talks about stress, as well as pride in her time-management skills:

I've perfected the art of doing two or three things at the same time. The one thing I really try to do is – if I'm interviewing clients, and I don't want to be fiddling with other things, but if the phone is ringing, or I'm put on hold – I'll usually have something next to me, so that I can start making notes or something like that.

Petra, on the other hand, implies that she feels inadequately trained. While her comments suggest pride in involving people in 'activity,' she perceives a lack of fit in relation to her professional team members:

I've had this activity background – this occupational therapy background; but so many of the things that I've found myself doing here, I'm not trained for.

Petra says that occupational therapists feel deficient but in other ways liberated by being different from professions that do not involve people in the ordinary activities of everyday life:

I think the liberating part is that I can go around and have these interactions with people in ways that people of other disciplines can't because there is such a gap between their training and someone else's. The breadth of occupational therapy allows therapists to close gaps between ourselves and people. We are not so different from them when it comes down to doing ordinary activities. We can relate to many people. We offer a bridge in our transitional work since we know something about the real work of people.

Rather than identify difference, deficiency or liberation in her work, Rasha told me that she tries to overcome her feelings of powerlessness by using her 'unique skills' as an occupational therapist:

I had to look at where my unique skills could be utilized the best. And also what I would like ... where my preferences were for enjoying my work.

Rasha also points to her difficulty in doing 'occupational therapy things,' given limited time and energy for the overall job:

I've been feeling overwhelmed by the number of requests to do occupational therapy things – particularly things like linking people to leisure interests ... so what I'm asking for is understanding from the rest of the team when I say no to some of your requests ... I am more assertive [as the team has suggested] and state my limits, but then I'm asked to take six more cases.

Carol struggles to organize part-time, trial work experiences for people in mental health services. She is responsible for locating and supervising people in hospital industries, such as food services or maintenance. When she approaches the designated supervisors of these units, she describes what people can do:

We try to give the supervisors information on someone without giving any real history or background of their illness or anything like that – everything is very confidential. If there's anything relating to their ability to work – for example, that they may need a time out, or that they may need a quiet area for working – we may say something about the amount of responsibility they are ready to take on. But we only give them information that's really needed.

Neva experiences tension surrounding the documentation of practice. As she talks about empowerment, she points to the problem of documentation connected with being part of a hospital,

because that keeps you quite attached to the medical model of stuff although you're trying to work with something that's very different ... the time you have to spend fulfilling hospital quality assurance and program kinds of stuff ... charting, statistics, all that kind of stuff. And also because there's a different kind of mind-set if you're doing that.

Britte reveals another aspect of tension by talking about the contradiction in extending practice beyond hospital facilities. Efforts to involve people in real life appear to be appreciated by the team but are financially unrecognized by the hospital:

I don't do it much. I do go out. I'm just not reimbursed for it. I get my pay for working. But I'm not given mileage. It's not recognized that I actually do it.

Britte articulates the belief that occupational therapy has potential to involve people in empowering ways. The dilemma, for Britte, is one of being 'not well developed':

The occupational therapy role in mental health is not well developed ... we're not very clear on the role ourselves.

Britte points to employment in a hospital setting as a source of tension:

Just the fact that I'm working here, and I'm working in [a hospital-based site] such as this, means that I'm working in contradiction to some of my values and beliefs in what I could be doing to empower people. I work here because this is where I can get paid. This is where things are established. But that's in contradiction to what I preach about people learning to be responsible for themselves in the community.

Mai perceives that there are 'major barriers' that limit professional involvement in advocacy, even though 'there's no regulation saying things have to be done this way or that way.'

It seems to me that the major barriers for occupational therapists, and maybe for other workers as well, are that a lot of what needs to be done is not within their own work environment, day-to-day environment. There's no regulation saying things have to be done this way or that way, but there are barriers in some of the broader things that we talked about – such as there being limits to the involvement you can have in advocating for changes that would make life easier for certain kinds of people. The barriers are more outside of the work situation, and yet they do affect your work.

Mai does not experience restriction from regulations in her immediate work situation, but rather from broader conflict-of-interest barriers that limit government employees from advocating for self-help, volunteer, or paid services that might be provided outside government.

In daily practice, the tension between enabling participation and caregiving manifests itself in juggling large caseloads and paperwork requirements, with little time to help people become involved in their own communities. Occupational therapists also experience difficulty in encouraging people to take on responsibility in their own lives, while simultaneously controlling decisions about their need for time out. A key aspect of the tension is illustrated by the inability to involve people in 'activities' when this approach does not fit with the work of other team members in mental health programs. The tension between participation and caregiving is also evident when occupational therapists attempt to guide people through the transition from hospital to community life, while also keeping track of them on behalf of psychiatrists and managers. Another aspect of the tension shows itself when occupational therapists involve people in simulation activities in hospitals rather than in the real occupations that have meaning in the communities where people live. Professionals who might see the need for services beyond their day-to-day work environment cannot advocate to expand community support services because this would be viewed as a conflict of interest.

In each occupational therapist's statement, quoted above, one can see that the experience of tension differs. My challenge was to discover how these experiences were interconnected examples of an *organized* tension related to empowerment. First, I needed to find out what was already known about empowerment and about empowerment issues particular to mental health services and occupational therapy.

What Is Known about Empowerment?[2,3]

Empowerment has become a trivialized buzz-word in North America. We talk about empowering students by educating them to think for themselves. Or we say that community residents are empowering themselves if they open community gardens where they can grow their own food. Legislation is said to be empowering if it enables single parents to collect support payments from absentee parents. Employers see themselves as empowering employees when they allow their workers to participate in decisions to make work more efficient. Sometimes empowerment is linked with those identified as *special-interest groups*. For instance, people with physical disabilities speak about empowerment as a foundation for independent living. Anti-poverty groups link their empowerment to their vision of social equity. Women and men who seek pay equity, not only for the same job but for work of equal complexity, talk about differing struggles for empowerment. Experiments with affirmative action are often described as opportunities for empowerment. Sometimes empowerment is talked about in terms of equal access to employment, housing, and other areas of life. Spiritual empowerment is equated with personal enlightenment and transformation. In addition, health promotion experts recognize that empowerment has a major influence on health.

If we listen carefully to the diverse views cited above, they reveal elements rather than the totality of empowerment. Each element is necessary, but insufficient on its own. Helping employees to feel better about their work, for instance, is not sufficient for empowerment, unless there are changes in the structure and organization of work; conversely, social change legislation does not empower single parents unless they perceive themselves as being empowered and act as such in everyday situations.

Psychological views about empowerment point to the importance of individuals *feeling* more powerful. Many organizations encourage individuals to participate in taking personal responsibility and making choices in order to feel empowered. This stance emphasizes the importance of developing feelings that one has power to influence life. A related, psychological interpretation of empowerment is taken by those who highlight the need to transform one's personal perspective on the power to change one's life. Here the focus is on individuals transforming *thoughts* about their feelings, sense of meaning, beliefs and values about being powerless or powerful in relation to others, and in particular situations. A perspective transformation occurs when people develop their self-understanding, self-esteem, resilience, and confidence so that they believe in and exert their own power. Processes of perspective transformation engage people in rethinking and reconceptualizing themselves in light of everyday experiences. There is optimism in creating perceptions of a more powerful self who is able to manage life with greater satisfaction and effectiveness. Psychological stories tap human agency: the power to get up and go, to pull ourselves up by the bootstraps, or to persevere in difficult circumstances. They point to the power of believing in ourselves and persisting resolutely towards our goals.

Some may view the *spirit*, more than feelings and thoughts, as a source of transformation. In theological terms, transformation lies in following the teachings of a powerful leader or god. Stories that highlight empowerment as a spiritual transformation tell about individuals who are guided through spiritual journeys towards new visions and experiences of spiritual power. Individuals are connected with a powerful life force that strengthens human agency and links humans with a divine will.

Psychological and theological perspectives on empowerment may also emphasize the importance of translating new-found feelings of power into everyday *action*, to actually *do* something to realize dreams of equality and justice. Empowerment may be equated with behaviours and actions such as assertiveness, good deeds, performance, function, and other ways of acting more powerful. North Americans, in particular, turn to all kinds of courses, workshops, and self-help approaches that promise them they will become empowered to deal with their employers, partners, parents, and others. Assertiveness is contrasted with aggression when there is an abuse of power, and passivity is viewed as dependence on the power of others. Whatever the approach, the emphasis in empowerment action is on sharing power collaboratively in what are often described as horizontal relationships, in contrast with hierarchical relations, in which some people control what others do.

To gain a fuller picture of empowerment, we need to supplement these *individualized* views with a *social* understanding that empowerment is more than just an individual experience of feeling good and behaving assertively. In fact, individualized conceptions of empowerment (personal, individual empowerment) implicitly lay blame on individuals who lack power. We are victimizing unempowered individuals if we say that they alone are the makers of their misfortunes. Since opportunities to feel good and behave assertively are determined by the structure and organization of society, we need to recognize that empowerment affects us all. If we acknowledge that empowerment has social elements, we begin to understand how empowerment forms a foundation for visionary ideas such as participatory democracy, collaborative partnerships, social equity, and the inclusion of all people in society regardless of ability, age, gender, race, social class, sexual orientation, or other forms of difference.

When we talk about the social elements of empowerment, then, we are talking about legislative, policy, financial, and organizational processes, and about the potential of these processes to create social equity. The social elements of empowerment include voting privileges being extended to women or people of African-American descent, minimum wage legislation, child labour laws, and affirmative action legislation. All of these initiatives promote empowerment by changing the opportunities for exercising power by various populations, whether or not these opportunities are taken up by individuals. In other words, a local government or nation-state can empower those who, by virtue of their limited skills, age, ethnicity, gender, or race, are vulnerable to exploitation. Legislation may not remove everyday, individual experiences of oppression or subordination, but it draws a line that publicly declares a society's ethical commitment to an empowerment minimum.

Sometimes the issue of governance – the political and organizational processes of governing – is raised in reference to empowerment. Processes of governance support empowerment when there are universal opportunities for people to vote, participate in public debates without fear of reprisal, and make choices about the organization of their communities and countries. An empowerment-based society would guarantee unobstructed communication and action for all citizens. Enlightenment and empowerment would be fostered through the debate of ideas and through public participation in all forms of decision making. Empowerment would progress when collaboration is incorporated into information gathering, decision making, and action on local, national, and international matters. For empowerment and social equity to occur, governance would ideally be organized to equalize opportunities for self-expression and action. An example of an existing equalizing governance practice in North America is the public financing of ramps for people in wheelchairs. It is the organization of policies and finances, not just idealism and rhetoric, that promote the empowerment of these people by providing the money, policies, and legislation needed to guarantee access to buildings regardless of ability.

When we recognize that empowerment has social elements, we can see the importance of governments organizing the *system* so that vulnerable people, including those who are different from what we call the norm, have the same opportunities as others. The system consists of those processes that are embedded in everyday *institutional* functions in any realm, from health services to transportation. The term institution does not refer here to a building. I am drawing on Dorothy Smith's reference to social institutions to mean organizational units that determine how we look after ourselves, attend to our health, work, play, educate our children, run businesses, help those in need, arrange transportation, and worship (Smith, 1987, 1990a, 1990b). In other words, the system produces the broad *social organization* of power. Although we experience the system in everyday situations, we are not fully conscious of social organization because power is organized outside the day-to-day experience of individuals. The system often feels anonymous and objective, but its policies, funding, legislation, and other elements are highly ideological. As Smith says, ideology is not merely a set of ideas; rather, ideology shapes the practical organization of knowledge and power through the textual and other methods used to govern everyday life. Of course, power can be exerted visibly through aggression, coercion, manipulation, or violence, but modern societies are more likely to organize power in the invisible processes that govern what we do. Modern societies organize knowledge so that the dominant methods of organization form what Smith (1987) calls a *ruling apparatus*. Certainly we need coordinating mechanisms to organize the complexities of modern society. None the less, invisible processes coordinate and control institutional functions such as health services, transportation, or social welfare. These institutions are coordinated so that very particular (not random) methods of organizing health, transportation, and welfare prevail. Other organizational processes are subordinated by defining them as irrelevant, frill, or alternative to mainstream, funded practices.

A topical example in Canada is health services. Health services fund organizational processes that support medicine's emphasis on the treatment of disease. Practices that promote health through everyday living, spirituality, or empowerment are subordinated if they do not fit the medical organization of health services. In Canada, the only health services funded by Canada's national health insurance program are those that are organized and controlled, directly or indirectly, by medical physicians. One can experience the medical ideology of health services in the types of health services that are funded, but the medical organization of health services occurs outside our everyday experience of visiting an occupational therapist, physician, or other health practitioner.

Overall, it seems that dynamic interactions between personal and social processes are what propel and energize empowerment. As individuals experience a transformation in their feelings and thoughts of power, they begin to act more powerfully in everyday situations; conversely, social processes that guarantee the routine, equitable sharing of power encourage individuals to feel, think, and act as citizens who can expect to share power. Because of this synergy, the empowerment of new groups does not mean that others must lose power; empowerment is a process and a social relation, not a finite or scarce commodity, or a quantifiable object with boundaries. Instead, empowerment is a generative process in which power grows for all as it is shared. In other words, there is no need to jostle or compete for empowerment, or to disempower others in order to become empowered. Of course, those whose power has been supported by the ruling apparatus will experience power differently if others gain power. Nevertheless, collaborative power is generated as hierarchical control and authority are dismantled.

This generative understanding of empowerment is what makes it a forward-looking process that transforms systems as well as individuals. Transformation, however, is a time-consuming and labour-intensive process of experimentation. The process is energized by ideas of hope, trust, generosity, and love, which sustain people through transformative change that may threaten or overwhelm them as they take on responsibility for sharing power. The energy for empowerment is fostered, in Freire's words, through a 'language of possibility' and a 'prophetic vision' that articulates a 'philosophy of hope' (1985, pp. xvi–xvii). Joan Kuyek (1990) describes the process of empowerment as fighting for hope.

If we think about the scope of empowerment that I have outlined here, should we dismiss the term because it has been trivialized? I think not. Empowerment is extremely important because it propels us to draw on a vision of fairness so that we transform everyday life in order to achieve *what might be or ought to be*. Moreover, critiques of empowerment are necessary because of the centrality of power in human existence; they encourage reflection, questioning, suspicion, and doubt about *what is* in order to energize us into changing today into a more equitable tomorrow. In addition, ethical practices that share power equitably need to be encouraged to bring enlightenment, transformation, health, and fairness into reality. It seems that empowerment is important to us all, whether our professional or management positions carry power or whether we lack power in our positions as students, community residents, employees, workers, people with disabilities, or people living in poverty. In the field of health promotion, empowerment is the foundation for self-help, public participation, and the development of community resources. Essentially, healthy public policy would make empowerment a basis of society.

These characteristics – a vision, a process of critique, participatory action, a power relation, an ethical commitment, a process of education and learning, a central force in human existence – make empowerment dynamic, far-reaching, and radical, but also essential for individuals and societies. Simply put, empowerment involves us all. Surely we should not cynically dismiss such compelling processes as trivial when they touch everyone. Empowerment is available to all who both are willing and have the opportunity to share power and material resources; it should be a positive experience if people realize their potential without oppressing others. Possibilities for enabling empowerment rest on a synergy and dynamism between individual and social processes that create a distributive, inclusive form of social justice.

Based on this broad view of empowerment and the practices observed in this study, we can say that *empowerment is a participatory process of learning to critique and transform individual feelings, thoughts, and actions, as well as the organization of society, so that power and resources can be shared equitably.*

Why Explore Empowerment in Mental Health Services?

Disability and Mental Health Problems[4]

Barriers to empowerment differ depending on whether inequalities are associated with gender, race, sexual orientation, ability, or other source of difference. People with disabilities historically have been among the most disempowered people. They have tended to be either sanctified as special or segregated out of fear and disgust, or because of their own inability to fit into mainstream society. Disability is a general term referring to limited ability, arising from physical, emotional, cognitive, learning, sensory, or other bodily impairments that place some people outside what are considered normal expectations for everyday performance. Impairment refers to pathology or dysfunction in bodily systems or parts, whereas handicap refers to a social limitation in housing, employment, or other life experience if society is not organized to include people with disabilities. The terms impairment, disability, and handicap have been differentiated to convey that people with impairments or disabilities do not need to be handicapped (World Health Organization, 1980).

Since the 1970s, much attention has been given to people defined as physically disabled, particularly public figures such as Canada's Rick Hansen. Such people are now able to participate more fully in regular society with the help of wheelchairs, technical aids, and architectural adaptations to buildings, streets, and transportation. People with physical disabilities have advanced their empowerment through personal transformation and through political, economic, and legal modifications. Changes in organization and governance have created opportunities for people with physical disabilities to gain employment, decent housing, and fairer access to sports and recreation. Their transformation has been helped enormously by technology and by the development of independent living centres and self-help groups.

In contrast, people diagnosed with long-lasting mental disorders have had far less success in participating in mainstream society. Such people continue to face negative social stigma and segregation. They experience powerlessness as both a symptom and consequence of a mental disorder, or what many now prefer to call a mental health problem. The shift in terminology is itself an attempt to destigmatize mental difficulties and to stop locating them solely in genetic, biochemical, or other biological causes. Such terminology reflects the view that oppressive social conditions aggravate or even cause some mental health problems, resulting in people experiencing a downward drift in social class. Regardless of their origin, mental health problems can reduce people's ability to think, feel, act, and organize. Long-standing mental health problems seriously interfere with everyday life. People with severe, persistent mental health problems are likely to live a marginalized existence with limited employment, housing, recreation, and other opportunities. Their mental health problems often undermine their potential as political actors and advocates for their own rights.

Unfortunately, feelings of powerlessness may be worsened by the process of psychiatric diagnosis and treatment. A diagnosis of mental disorder can provide invaluable treatment information, but it can also isolate and victimize those so diagnosed as diseased and undesirable in ordinary society. The individualizing process of psychiatric diagnosis structures treatment to attend primarily to biological elements and to leave the social elements of mental health problems for attention by other institutions, such as social services, education, and employment. Many critiques have highlighted problems related to psychiatric diagnosis, but mental health problems are real. Furthermore, those who experience these problems often need both individual attention and help in advocating for social change.

Given their vulnerability and experiences of powerlessness, people with severe mental health problems offer us an important social gauge. If we look at the services organized to help these people, we have one way of assessing our commitment to empowerment and thus to justice. We can see if our institutions are actually encouraging its less powerful citizens to become empowered.

Mental Health Professionals[5]

Numerous books have explored the experiences of people living with a mental health problem, or critique mental health services from the insider perspective of patients. Outside researchers have also developed a variety of critiques of mental health services. In these works we are often told that professionals dominate and disempower patients and that those who are frequent or long-standing recipients of mental health services lack power in society. Their lack of power is visibly observable in their poverty, their discrimination at work and in neighbourhoods, and their marginalization in communities. De-institutionalization has not released these people from professional control; rather, it has changed the way control is exercised over them.

This book takes a different approach. I am writing from the point of view of a mental health professional. Analyses of medicine and law have shown the dominant and patriarchal character of these professions. Other professions, especially those practised mainly by women, show a more contradictory character: good intentions become caught up in bureaucracy. What seem like positive helping strategies often subordinate people's own experience to professional expertise, so that professionals end up in positions of dominance, even when working for and with those who are oppressed. Moreover, the hierarchical organization of state-managed health and welfare services has been identified more with dependency than empowerment. In mental health services, professionals may be interested in enabling empowerment, but the state expects mental health professionals to control deviance in order to ensure the safety of citizens and to preserve existing social and economic patterns of living. Given this contradictory position, critiques of psychology, social work, and health promotion have already asked if professionals can truly help others to become empowered. From the mountain of literature on professional dominance, I knew that I would find many constraints for professionals who want to enable people with mental health problems to become empowered.

Nevertheless, it seemed important to understand how empowerment works from a professional standpoint if professionals are to learn to practise *reflexively*, in the words of George Smith (1994), who examined health reform in Ontario in the 1990s. With awareness of their participation in ruling institutions, professionals might reduce their dominance and become translators, transmitters, facilitators, and activists who work with and on behalf of the people they want to help.

Occupational Therapy[6]

In explaining my interest in empowerment and professional mental health services, I now come to my occupational therapy perspective. Occupational therapy offers an intriguing window for looking at empowerment. This profession defines itself as client-centred in that we intend to enable people to choose, organize, and perform those occupations they find useful or meaningful in their environment (Canadian Association of Occupational Therapists [CAOT], 1997). Occupational therapy is often presented, by occupational therapists and others, as a medically oriented profession, striving to be, with medicine, part of the dominant ruling apparatus. Yet the underlying intention of being client-centred and focusing on everyday occupations is to enable all people, including those with disability, old age, or social disadvantage, to become empowered by changing their functional potential and their environment so that they can live useful and meaningful lives. Many occupational therapists work with individuals who have a medical diagnosis, but we also report almost a century of activist involvement in changing conditions in workplaces, homes, schools, and public buildings with those whose everyday lives are limited by aging or social disadvantage as well as disability.

While occupational therapists are best known for our work with those who have physical disabilities, the profession emerged out of the experience of 'occupation workers' who encouraged insane people to engage, for healing as well as sustenance, in farming, laundry, handcrafts, and other occupations that were part of life in nineteenth-century workhouses and asylums. 'Occupational work' was later organized as 'occupational therapy' to enable wounded soldiers to return to work or learn to live with disabilities acquired during the First World War. Today, around 20 per cent of occupational therapists work in mental health services or psychosocial programs with those who have a physical disability (CAOT, 1996a).

How Does an Institutional Ethnography Explore Empowerment?

Some people try to measure selected characteristics of empowerment, or they seek to understand personal experiences of empowerment. Instead, this book shows how empowerment actually works by asking questions such as: What does empowerment look like in everyday situations? What are the empowering and disempowering forms of organization that determine the potential for empowerment in everyday situations? How are everyday situations and organizational processes interconnected to produce the routine, taken-for-granted organization of particular institutions, such as mental health services?

To answer these questions, I used Canadian sociologist Dorothy Smith's theory and method of *institutional ethnography* (Smith, 1987, 1990a, 1990b). Institutional ethnography is a materialist theory and method that Smith developed from five main sources: (1) her experiences as a woman in academia and society; (2) her use of ethnomethodology to question taken-for-granted social practices; (3) feminist ideas about work processes; (4) the phenomenology of everyday experience articulated by Alfred Schutz (1967) and Berger & Luckmann (1967); and (5) Marx's German ideology, which describes the hierarchical relations of power that are reproduced by labour in the material conditions of capitalism.

'Materialist' methods analyse what people actually do in the physical, social, and other conditions of real life. It follows that institutional ethnographies analyse the ways in which organizational processes produce a generalized way of living in the everyday world, regardless of differences in particular individuals and circumstances. Furthermore, the analysis shows how power is socially organized by a ruling apparatus. In other words, this type of analysis reveals the ruling relations in a particular institution from a standpoint that begins with lived experience, such as the tension described at the beginning of this chapter.

Beginning with a Disjuncture

An institutional ethnography starts with what is called a standpoint *in* the everyday world. This standpoint differs from experimental research, in which one attempts to take an objective, outsider's point of view. It also differs from interpretive research, which may present an insider's or outsider's analysis of subjective feelings, meanings, and perceptions of human experience. Instead, the institutional ethnographer listens to and observes experiences of tension as a starting point for tracing the actual activities and conditions of the everyday world to the organizational processes that invisibly rule that experience.

Smith refers to experiences of tension as a disjuncture, line of fault, or bifurcation of consciousness. A disjuncture may exist between what is experienced and what is officially known (measured, recorded, analysed) about that experience; or the disjuncture may be a contradiction between what is intended and what actually happens, between vision and reality. A bifurcated consciousness exists when one is conscious of everyday experiences while remaining unconscious of the taken-for-granted, invisible organization of power that controls and coordinates the everyday world.

In a state of bifurcated consciousness, occupational therapists often perceive that practice is misunderstood and has undeveloped potential. Everyday practice – for instance, enabling people to shop and cook meals – is misunderstood to be simple and common sense unless the complex reasoning and broad, underlying purpose are explained. Much of the complexity goes unrecorded, while performance measurements and simple behaviourial changes are noted. Moreover, the potential to enable people to become empowered in living useful and meaningful lives is hampered by insufficient funding, inadequate time to offer more than technical approaches, and other features that occupational therapists know from experience limit what they can do. When asked, occupational therapists innately know how everyday practice works, but we have been unaware of our professional power, and there have been no institutional analyses that explicitly show how the organization of power in mental health and other services determines what occupational therapists can do, or how the myriad tensions experienced in practice are produced by fundamental contradictions in the social organization of occupational therapy. Without a full understanding of the routine, institutional organization of practice, occupational therapists' potential to enable empowerment is rarely realized in actual practice, true occupational therapy being largely a vision, not a reality.

As I proceeded with the ethnography, I began to hear different aspects of the tension between the complexity I observed and heard described, and official accounts of practice; moreover, there was a considerable gap between occupational therapists' intentions of being client-centred, and the reality of practice. You have already heard how the occupational therapists in this study experienced tension.

Describing the Everyday World

As I describe my approach to collecting data, I encourage you to picture a funnel. Data collection began broadly then gradually narrowed (funnelled) until there was saturation. In an institutional ethnography, saturation occurs when sufficient data are collected to record how everyday practice actually works within an institutional framework. To discover occupational therapists' experiences of disjuncture, I undertook the rather arduous task of describing the everyday world of occupational therapy. This is the first of what Smith calls the *analytic processes* of institutional ethnography. I collected data using three methods that are common to any type of ethnography: participant observation, interview, and documentary review. Each process is analytic in that it shapes the investigation consistent with the theoretical framework of institutional ethnography.

This book is based on six months of field study with the seven occupational therapists whom I have called Jill, Petra, Rasha, Carol, Neva, Britte, and Mai. Each occupational therapist was in a different site, selected so that I would see how occupational therapy works in day programs, out-patient services, or community mental health services – all of which are services designed to keep people out of hospital – in the four provinces of Atlantic Canada: New Brunswick, Newfoundland, Nova Scotia, and Prince Edward Island. My selection ensured that at least one site was in each province. I added the regional criterion to protect the occupational therapists' anonymity. Anonymity would be extremely difficult to protect in the small occupational therapy and mental health community of this region if I had studied only one occupational therapist's experience or the experiences of a few occupational therapists in any one province. Without these multiple sites, it would be too easy to read the data as an evaluation of each occupational therapist's practice.

I began by collecting data in the first two sites for eight and six weeks respectively, full time (eight hours a day) in each site. During the six weeks after gathering data on Petra's practice at what I will call Penrose day program (all are called day programs to protect their identity), I developed and presented my initial analytic ideas for response from Petra. At this point the analysis offered reflections. For instance, I reflected on Petra's involvement in running groups while also being responsible for organizing a workshop and kitchen, as well as outings in the community. Additional reflections were incorporated and presented for Rasha's comments after I collected data in Rosehill day program. An example of additional reflections was that Rosehill's program facilities and schedules emphasized more group work than I had seen at Penrose. My third stop was for one week with Neva in New Garden day program. Here I noted that the program philosophy and facility encouraged people to participate in weekly meetings, cook meals for each other, do maintenance, and complete the clerical work associated with running the program.

On reflection, I decided that I still had not seen the full scope of occupational therapy's mental health work. I took a few weeks to review my notes, forward my research proposal for ethics review in four more sites, and catch up on transcribing observations and interviews. When approval was received from Bayview day program, I spent almost a week with Britte. Britte's practice included more administrative duties than did the practices of Petra, Rasha, or Neva. After spending time at Bayview, I went for a few days each to record practice under differing managerial lines of authority at Jackson Heights day program with Jill, and Clearcove day program with Carol. Through my visits to these sites, I was able to see differences as well as similarities in the ways that occupational therapists decide on goals and programs when they are singularly responsible to an occupational therapy departmental manager as opposed to being doubly responsible in what managers call *matrix management*; for example, in Clearcove day program, Carol was responsible for personnel matters to an occupational therapy departmental manager, while also being responsible for program decisions to the coordinator of the mental health day program. Finally, I visited Mai at Merrivale day program. At this point I wanted to clarify differences in Mai's emphasis on working with individuals rather than groups. By this time I had documents as well as participant observation and interview data from the first six sites and interview data from my visit with Mai. From the broad sweep where data collection had begun, I had funnelled my enquiries to a point of saturation where I was seeing no new variations or contradictions.

Tracing Social Processes

The second analytic process in an institutional ethnography involves tracing the social processes that connect the work being studied with the work of others – in this case, the policies, procedures, classifications, legislation, statistics, and other social processes that coordinate and control occupational therapy. These social processes are organizational in that they routinely organize what can be done in everyday practice. Through a back-and-forth method of exploration, I traced connections between what occupational therapists do and the documentation and other processes that govern that work.

For instance, I noted that occupational therapists sometimes help people to cook in kitchens. To trace this observation, I noted who else works in kitchens, then I asked and read how this work is reported to others in official situations such as team meetings and public presentations. Interviews were used to ask how the place, time, and general plans for the meal were decided. Who did this work of deciding? How was the kitchen paid for? Who purchased and monitored kitchen supplies? How was the work of guiding meal planning and preparation documented within the time management and management information systems used in mental health services? My observations and interviews determined what documents were reviewed. I looked at schedules and brochures on bulletin boards to see if they explained why meal planning and preparation are part of these programs. I also reviewed schedules, activity plans, and policy and procedure documents on groups, accountability, liability legislation, decision making, responsibility, quality assurance, risk and crisis management, and confidentiality to find out how occupational therapists' work in kitchens and other places is organized in Canada's provincial and national systems of mental health services.

The process of analysing connections extends from data collection into data management and the early stages of data analysis. After the completion of data collection in the seven sites, I coded data as a way of distilling and grouping occupational therapy work processes. Sorting was done by grouping data on actual work, not by clustering data into interpretive themes such as *choice.* In essence, the codes used to sort data in an institutional ethnography describe the segments of everyday practice. Material is coded, then examined to see how various everyday activities are interrelated, such as connecting the data on occupational therapists facilitating meal preparation with the data on records of people engaged in meal preparation.

I coded my notes by converting transcripts of observations and interviews for use with ETHNOGRAPH, a computer software package. Since occupational therapy involves a wide range of work processes, there were many codes for the work of coaching people in groups, speaking to community and city officials, reporting at medical rounds, and so forth. For example, one group of codes described the work of organizing weekly program activities in connection with other professionals, particularly psychiatrists and psychologists, who have generally defined the broader framework for day programs. Then I grouped the work of involving people in actual program activities under codes such as 'leading individual and group sessions about the self and everyday life,' 'helping people to find community support groups,' 'investigating employment, housing, and social recreation programs,' and 'determining regulations for financial assistance.' When occupational therapists' administrative work was coded, I could see how occupational therapy is also connected with mental health services management. These connections are reproduced every time occupational therapists prepare budgets for supplies used in everyday activities, document time in a workload measurement system, participate in case management, and record data on numbers and types of cases seen.

Displaying Ideology and Objectified Management

The third process of an institutional ethnography extends the analysis to display the ideological character of the organizational processes that coordinate and control the work done by an institution. Described here is the social organization of knowledge in a particular institution. It is at this stage that we can see how ideology is practised in everyday situations: visible are organizational processes that are embedded in actual activities in the material conditions of everyday life, while also being 'external to the local and particular places of one's bodily existence' (Smith 1987, p. 84) and 'generalizers of actual local experience' (p. 154). These are the material practices of ideology that 'coordinate and codetermine the worlds, activities, and experiences of people entered into them at different points' (p. 134) – that is, how particular, differing instances of practice take on generalized organizational patterns.

The material practice of ideology is particularly visible in the texts of an institution. As used by Smith, the word *text* refers to a wide variety of documentary media that create an account of or otherwise represent experience (Smith, 1990a). My textual analysis included the documents described above, as well as statistics, professional textbooks, information management processes, presentation overheads used to describe the program to others, and so on. These texts helped me to see the disjuncture between objectified knowledge and the subjective knowledge of occupational therapists' actual experience. I examined textual 'facts' as objects that form an account of what is textually 'known' about people and work processes (p. 104), looking to see how accounts of occupational therapy both display and organize the 'objectified forms' that have been used by mental health services to coordinate and control occupational therapy 'through the text' (p. 4). It was fascinating to see how routine documentary activities, like filling in admission forms, are used to control decision making in the objectified management of occupational therapists and people with mental health problems.

Objectified management refers simply to the management of textual objects using scientific methods that do not require face-to-face personal contact (Cassin, 1990). Since objectified management relies on the objectified methods of empirical science, it is sometimes called 'scientific management.' The processes of objectified management require, at the outset, the objectification of people as cases or units. Therefore, my analysis examined how occupational therapists and the people with whom occupational therapists work are conceptualized and categorized in mental health services, then coordinated and controlled through textual facts about these categories rather than through face-to-face supervision.

As an illustration of how objectified or scientific management operates, *admission* and *case management* in mental health services are real activities in occupational therapists' day-to-day work. These are textual processes that transform people into cases or units (giving each a number), and their experiences of admission and case management into numbers of cases (also known as caseloads). The amounts of time spent with each case are recorded to create data that are analysed in management information systems as part of the production of conceptual objects known as 'accountability' and 'total quality management.' The textual processes of admission and case management stabilize and create a conceptual order out of the disorder that is subjectively known in the day-to-day contacts between professionals and the people who are seeking access to and guidance from mental health services. These processes are ideological because they are organized to provide data on numbers of cases per diagnostic category of the mental disorders that have been defined by psychiatrists, and the numbers of cases that can be managed in day programs by particular numbers and types of professional and other staff. Admission, case management, and other textual processes create a *documentary reality*, that is, a set of textual facts that are used to account for the work accomplished in mental health services, and to guide it through policies and other documents. Interconnecting documents form the ruling apparatus of mental health services and create an *organizational impregnability* (Smith's words) since ruling cannot be attributed to any of the individuals who work in or use mental health services. Selected facts are used to make decisions that are difficult to trace to actual people, yet actual people have created textual forms and facts, from public relations materials to management information systems. They create facts to interpret activities in ways that are relevant to the work of those who are dominant in an institution. Activities that are not considered relevant to an institutional function are not officially recorded and thus are rendered largely invisible and powerless to shape the practices within that institution. Whereas admission and case management seem to be objective, unbiased processes, they are ideologically biased because the types of people who can be admitted, and the processes that follow admission, are organized primarily to support the medical work of psychiatrists.

The analysis of ideology in an institutional ethnography requires time, reading, and thought, particularly since this method generates a large, complex database. My observation notes are full of conversations and actions as mundane as occupational therapists speaking to people at water fountains about their bus fare to and from programs. It took a long period of reading, thinking, and reflecting before I began to see how talking about buses at the water fountain displays interconnections between diverse work processes. I gradually realized that asking individuals about their transportation connects occupational therapy with the institutional process of individual case management. Individual cases are often monitored by asking people about their lives during the course of a day program. The work is not always done by sitting in an office or by officially interviewing people.

A conversation about bus tickets at a water fountain is quite deliberate if a person has a goal such as 'become more independent in taking public transportation.' I became aware of the official underpinning to this water fountain conversation when I saw the occupational therapist write about transportation on the person's health record. Notes about bus tickets might be cross-referenced in individual health records to a list of assessed problems, such as 'feeling too anxious to interact with people in public places,' or 'need to contact social services to get more bus tickets.'

On reflection, I realized that these seemingly brief documentary notes of a problem, goal, and progress are used to make a profession's work accountable for individual case management, the mechanism adopted to coordinate and control the work done by mental health services. After a while I became conscious that giving out bus tickets also provides a concrete example of a material practice in which occupational therapy intersects with social welfare. Occupational therapists are administering the face-to-face philanthropic work of providing special transportation allowances to people whom the state recognizes as having special needs.

I also struggled to recognize instances of empowerment among many examples of disempowerment. With an emphasis on critique, the tendency is to concentrate on ways in which a ruling apparatus submerges, subordinates, or otherwise overrules empowering practices. I had to remind myself that agency creates in us the potential to resist what is. This realization gave me optimism and hope to name positive instances as moments of empowerment, moments in which there is resistance to the established system, which so often overrules empowerment. At times, drafts of my analysis sounded idealistic and uncritical, with tensions receding into the background while glimpses of empowerment gained excessive prominence. At other times, descriptions of constraints on empowerment seemed to obliterate the glimpses. Gradually, I understood how professional practice is ruled by the ways in which mental health services conceptualize and categorize people, account for everyday practice, organize decision making, manage safety, and promote change.

As the analysis progressed, I grouped my coded material under the six core features of empowerment that are inherent in occupational therapy. For example, I had initially grouped evidence of the actual activities of categorizing people's mental health problems under a descriptive code called DIAG (various actions that are part of diagnosing people). Now DIAG has been grouped with data coded as REFER (the work of handling referrals to mental health services), ASSESS (assessing people's reasons for using mental health services), and ADMIT (completing forms required before people can participate in mental health services). When grouped together, these data describe the work that is known as admission and assessment, and that is coordinated and controlled using the psychiatric diagnostic categories of mental disorder. Diagnoses related to categories of mental disorder control who can participate and what participation (involvement) or caregiving is encouraged. Through this type of tracing, I began to see how participation and caregiving depend on ideological, organizational processes that rule what can be done.

Finally, I realized that six features of empowerment are present *in* occupational therapy, at times supported but often overruled by the routine organization of adult mental-health day programs. The order of features described in each chapter will lead you to discover, as I did, how empowerment and barriers to empowerment are organized. We will first look at participation, because this feature is apparent the moment one enters the world of mental health services. We will then explore possibilities and constraints for individual and social action, collaborative decision making, learning through simulations or real experiences, risk taking, and social inclusiveness. Each chapter begins with what is considered to be 'ideal' for empowerment, then proceeds to show how good intentions are consistently overruled by processes used to organize mental health services. Since institutional ethnographies map out the social organization of knowledge in everyday life, they provide a blueprint for change. To that end, chapter 8 offers reflections on possible action if we wish to enable those with little power to become empowered.

Ethical Issues

Before I leave this overview of institutional ethnography, a word on ethics is in order. A growing number of researchers, particularly those using qualitative methods such as institutional ethnography, are emphasizing that ethics are not only a preliminary procedure, but are also an integral part of the research process to ensure that those who are the subject of research are not exploited. Mine was not a participatory research project in that I designed the study, collected data, and take responsibility for the final analysis. However, I could not have proceeded without occupational therapists' participation in all ethics, entry, and field relations until the analysis was complete.

Entry began with the first telephone call to the occupational therapist in each site selected. All occupational therapists agreed to participate in the research. I arranged informal agreement with each occupational therapist not by letter but by personal contact. Thankfully, each therapist supported and often facilitated submission of my proposal to the site-appropriate professional, administrative, and hospital research ethics review personnel.

In each site, mental health professionals, managers, and ethical reviewers were all consulted before the research was approved. To avoid misinterpretations, sites requested that people with mental health problems not sign consent forms so that it would be clear that I was researching occupational therapy, not those known as patients. On site, occupational therapists attended to people's rights to know about research being conducted in their presence, even though they were not research subjects. Anyone present had the right to ask me not to observe situations that involved them or to read records in which they would be seen interacting with the occupational therapist whose work I was analysing. Therefore I was constantly introduced by occupational therapists saying something like: 'Liz is following me to find out what I do. But you have the right to ask her not to come into this interview or to be part of the group. There is no penalty to you if you decide to say no.'

I was welcomed to observe all activities except a few discussions about sexual matters. People were wonderfully open to my presence and generally called me 'The Shadow.' The occupational therapists deserve tremendous credit for putting up with my prying eye; I followed them virtually everywhere.

Ensuring Rigour

The description of an institutional ethnography would not be complete without attention to questions about the rigour of this type of research. Rigour in quantitative research is judged by the research design, and by the validity and reliability of measurement and analytic procedures. In contrast, rigour in an institutional ethnography lies largely in clearly translating its theory and method into the research design and analysis. I am presenting my analysis as a true story: you are about to read an account of the actual activities of real people in real practice situations; you will also read how these activities are actually coordinated and controlled in mental health services. I have taken considerable trouble to describe how I collected and analysed data so that you know that you are reading about real situations rather than my personal impressions or interpretation of mental health services. You already know my standpoint for analysing power, ideology, social relations, and social organization.

In order to ensure that my argument fully accounts for the data, I reread and reflected on the uncoded database. Throughout the three analytic processes, I alternated rereading and thinking, regrouping coded material, and so on until I gradually focused the analytic points and the overall argument. All data are accounted for. I have tried to acknowledge any contradictions that would change the analysis. Initial analytic ideas went through many stages of refinement and change, not only as intellectual processes but as a physical process of revisiting the data and literature. Review of a draft analysis by the seven occupational therapists served as a check not only on confidentiality but also on the rigour in acknowledging similarities, differences, and contradictions. The main point they emphasized was that people's long-standing mental difficulties, as well as organizational processes, present barriers to their empowerment.

Generalizability

One last point is that this analysis displays broad generalizing social relations that organize practice within an institution. There is no intention to be generalizable in the statistical sense or in the conceptualization of a grand, generalized theory of society. Instead, the analysis reveals how institutional processes are ideological 'generalizers of actual local experience' (Smith, 1987, p. 154). This means that mental health services are characterized by generalizable power relations despite the diversity of practitioners, service users, and situations.

I will describe occupational therapy's mental health work in Atlantic Canada. However, mental health services are organized within Canada's national health system; thus, one can generalize the analysis to occupational therapy in mental health services across the country. The organizational features of mental health services are largely found in all professional mental health work in Canada, and to a large extent around the world. This generalizability is present because most mental health services are similarly organized. In fact, you will find many similarities to the social organization of power in all health services, education, welfare, and many other institutions. In essence, the analysis of occupational therapy illustrates how power and empowerment work in the industrialized societies of the late twentieth century.

2

Objectifying Participants

Empowerment has been described as a *participatory* process, meaning that it involves people as participants. We participate in life by activating mind, body, and spirit in the particular circumstances of our everyday lives. As long as we have breath to speak, muscles to move, or a spirit to express our beliefs, we can choose whether to participate in being disempowered or empowered. We cannot be empowered by others if we choose to be disempowered, nor will we participate actively if we choose to be passive or dependent. It follows that we involve others in empowerment by enabling their participation and by organizing possibilities for their participation. I discovered how the organization of power in mental health services determines participation by looking particularly at two processes: *assessment* and *admission.* I began to see how these processes objectify those who could be active participants.

Inviting Participation

We invite people to participate by valuing their worth, dignity, and rights, regardless of difference in mind, body, spirit, and circumstances – that is, regardless of disability, age, gender, class, or other characteristic. Moreover, every human can participate in some way because we can all exercise some degree of choice and exert some control even in the most debilitating or oppressive situations. For instance, those who are severely paralysed can exert control by directing others to help, visit, organize their schedule or otherwise interact with them as they wish; those who are hallucinating can choose whether or not to eat; when they are not hallucinating, they can declare their wishes on medication or other issues to those whom they trust when caregiving is needed.

To invite participation by individuals or groups is to be person-centred, and to be person-centred is to adopt particular concepts about people, three of which are highlighted here: humanism, autonomy, and an ethic of equality.

Humanism is a belief that takes human experience (rather than a god or encompassing power) as the starting point for knowledge of the self and the world. Humanism challenges notions that humans are merely constituents of social groups. People are viewed as holistic beings who have latent mental, physical, and spiritual power for integrating subjective experience into action. The implication is that people are active beings with agency to shape their lives, while also being shaped by the society in which they live. People can choose how to participate individually or collectively in their lives, even if choice is confined. We can make choices about our physical, social, cultural, legal, economic, and other circumstances if the opportunity is present to do so. Therefore, people have the inherent potential to change their individual experience, as well as to improve the conditions of their lives.

When liberated, such as by education, this latent power enables people to exercise freedom of choice and to take individual and collection action. Humanism refutes beliefs such as behaviourism, determinism, and nihilism for their devaluing of human potential and for reducing human existence to those elements that respond to scientific measurement. Instead, humanism draws on idealism, existentialism, and pragmatism, which celebrate the worth and capacity of all persons to be active participants in society.

Humanism is related to the concept of autonomy. Autonomy is generated in one's unique subjective expertise and capacity to think, act, and interact in a socially organized world. Because the potential for autonomy is socially circumscribed, autonomy grows when individual thought, action, and interaction are valued. Like humanism, the concept of autonomy directs us to recognize the potential agency in each of us to participate. Unfortunately, beliefs in humanism and autonomy are often used to support the overpowering individualism of Western societies, particularly in the United States. The emphasis on individualism makes many forget about the potential of economic, social, political, physical, and organizational conditions to foster or limit autonomy, and thus empowerment.

We need a third concept to understand our potential to participate in the process of empowerment: an ethic of equality. If we recognize that all people have the potential to participate as long as they are alive, it follows that all people ought to have equal opportunity to participate in society, including the power to participate in sharing power and resources. In practical terms, empowerment involves us all as equal 'persons,' the term used to confer legislated entitlement or 'personhood.' An ethic of equality underpins the commitment to confer personhood on all people regardless of difference. Equity in granting personhood entitles everyone to have equal opportunity to participate, in some way, in work, and to live decently, enjoy themselves, and belong to their communities, if they so choose.

If we are to invite people to participate in their empowerment, then we need to do more than encourage people to speak up in meetings. We need to liberate their potential to participate in the kind of education that guides people to think, act, and create both meaning and opportunity in their personal lives and their communities. This means educating people to exercise their autonomous *active power* in everyday life, and also educating them to organize society so that everyone has opportunities to participate. For example, one might educate individuals to participate in employment while also educating them to organize policies, budget priorities, and legislation that support new employment initiatives.

Inviting Participation in Everyday Practice

The occupational therapists in this study all work with people who have experienced mental difficulties ranging from confusion and distorted feelings to outright delusions. Some people have problems that last weeks or months; others have had years of difficulty living in ordinary communities. Whether or not the causes are social or biological, the mental difficulties they face are real, and include shortened concentration span, tangential thinking, uncertain decision making, variable and sometimes unpredictable emotional control and mood swings, heightened anxiety, and varying ability to organize daily life. Common among these people are experiences of feeling lethargic, unmotivated, distracted, confused, disjointed, out of touch with reality, terrified, infuriated, elated, and a host of other emotions that are so intense or unpredictable that they disrupt everyday life. They have experienced temporary or long-lasting disruptions that have undermined or altered their potential to participate in life and to choose courses of action.[1]

Yet the potential to participate remains because they are thinking, feeling, acting humans. Given the fluctuating nature of some mental difficulties, many experience periods when their potential to participate in life is fully present. Although mental difficulties may undermine or alter participation, my first impression in observing all seven occupational therapists was that people with mental health problems are strongly encouraged to participate as much as possible. When I asked what the people who attend these programs are called, the occupational therapists explained that they deliberately recognize them as active participants and refer to them, whenever possible, as clients or consumers rather than patients. The programs based on the psychosocial rehabilitation clubhouse philosophy go a step further by officially defining participants as members.[2]

You can observe people participating with occupational therapists in the work called *assessment*. Assessment in mental health services involves gathering information during sessions described as *initial*, *intake*, *screening*, *preliminary*, *pre-assessment*, or *trial* assessments. Mental health day programs are located in hospitals or in houses funded by hospitals. Even in hospital-based programs, assessment occurs in a space that is designed to simulate participation in ordinary life. If you are expecting a hospital look when you enter one of these programs, you will be taken aback. Health *care* is delivered to people who are lying down, sitting, or walking around. While caregiving is usually provided in bedrooms and testing done in professionally controlled laboratories, mental health day program professionals may start their assessment in offices and interview rooms, where people are asked about their current participation in everyday life. There are no professional uniforms, nor is anyone wearing hospital gowns. In fact, staff and those attending programs may be wearing cooks' hats and aprons, mechanics' overalls, carpenters' aprons, exercise clothes, business outfits, or casual everyday clothes as they participate in the work of these programs.

Where assessment occurs in old renovated houses, participation seems even more like active involvement than in specially designed hospital space. From both the outside and inside, these houses resemble residences. Inside they look like homes or offices in which people have established businesses. In the renovated houses, a kitchen, living room, and bathroom are being used by what looks like family members who are completing various ordinary life tasks. Otherwise, the place looks like a business, with a cafeteria for members and various work rooms. Some programs look like professional counselling offices, but the group rooms are often supplemented by a kitchen and various areas for completing projects or playing games. Some of the rooms are used for collating papers at tables, typing on computers, xeroxing, using sewing machines, packing boxes, and various other activities typical of office work. There may be a workshop with a table saw, drill press, anvil, wrenches, and other tools. Tools are in various states of use as people participate in building bird houses, fixing kitchen appliances, constructing Christmas tree ornaments, and so on. Even more than in hospital-based programs, space and time seem to be organized so that assessment is a process of seeing and hearing how people exert their autonomy and power to participate. The occupational therapists make a point of not only asking people what they can do, but observing participation as they cook in kitchens, sit in discussion groups, water plants, clean the program area, complete clerical tasks, make handcrafts, fix appliances in workshops, have coffee in lounges, and generally engage in the ordinary activities of everyday life.

Time also seems to be organized for participation. The occupational therapists and other staff make notes on who participated, what was done, and how participation worked out in various morning and afternoon events from Monday to Friday. Posted schedules invite people to read and follow them. From 6 to 30 people, some regulars and some sporadic attenders, generally show up each day and participate with the occupational therapists, other professionals, and the program secretary.

There is tremendous overlap and variation in the division of work among the mental health professionals in these programs; nevertheless, I found the occupational therapists to be particularly noticeable in a wide range of assessment opportunities. For instance, one day I observed Neva in the kitchen. As Lech walked in and said that he had some Polish recipes, Neva replied:

That would be great if you'd bring in a Polish recipe. We'd love to have a day of special recipes ... when you're chef, you can cook us a Polish meal. [Neva looks over at Sue and John making cream soup for a lunch dish] ... here, it's lumpy. You can use this whisk. [Neva then goes over to the oven to take out muffins and speaks to Ted] ... there, the oven is ready for your cake [turning back to Hal and Mack] ... do you guys know how to take out muffins? Don't be afraid to go right around [Neva demonstrates how to use a knife then takes a sip of the cream soup] ... mmm this tastes wonderful.

Neva is not providing service to waiting customers. She may conceptualize that people are holistic, autonomous, worthy beings, and she actually participates with them as active people who have their own interests and history. Neva is assessing participation in spaces and schedules that are made for participation in ordinary life events.

The occupational therapists appear to expect people to participate in their own assessment, starting with a classic occupational therapy question: How would you describe a typical day? The question is directed to the present (today? this week? in the last month?) and the past (over the last year? differences between this week and a year ago?). I was told that by asking when and where people are active, occupational therapists discern the dynamic, temporal, and spatial nature of people's participation in everyday life as autonomous active agents. These and other questions recognize that people have the power to be active in their daily lives despite their difficulties. Questions like these invite participation by active investigators whose subjective knowledge, no matter how distorted or frenzied, forms the basis of their own assessment.

This type of initial interview may raise questions for fifteen minutes to an hour. Thereafter an occupational therapist observes and talks to people in any part of the program. People are asked to compare their participation in the program with their participation in life outside the program. People are also engaged in everyday situations like cooking to observe how active they really are. Moreover, they are invited to reflect on their own participation through questions that relate their actions in the program space and time to their participation in real life.

If you observe for a while, you can see an interesting facet of this work. There are attempts to shift people's thinking away from their diagnostic symptoms and toward their power to participate in real life. Petra's initial interview with Carl shows how this happens.

Petra It seems that the last time you were here, you latched on to your diagnosis. Our concern in here is: what are you going to do about it?

Carl I was ready to do something about it six months ago. But I only got the diagnosis three months after I was here.

Petra It seems very important to you to have that label. I know that's important to some people but other people just know their problems and try to do something about them without worrying what label they have. What's happening with your day besides work?

Carl I'm just at home part of the time. That's part of the problem. I'm not doing anything. I'm not very independent.

Petra How could you be more independent?

Carl I could be married, have kids, have my own place.

Petra Those are the big ones. What about day to day? For instance, who does the cooking at home?

Petra listens to Carl's concern with his diagnosis but shifts the discussion from the diagnosis to his ability to participate in everyday life. She talks about 'being more independent' and makes the concept concrete by asking 'What's happening with your day besides work?' As Carl continues to theorize about marriage, children, and a home, Petra brings Carl back to day-to-day participation by asking 'What about day to day?' and 'Who does the cooking at home?' Petra later explained to me that she was asking about Carl's active involvement in life, recognizing that he is an active person with the capacity to change and improve his situation. She is also educating Carl to think about himself as an active participant in shaping his life. This assessment process educates Carl to understand his potential for participating in broad-ranging occupations even though he is unemployed and has a psychiatric diagnosis. Information is then recorded in Carl's health record as evidence of what is called *home management, personal care,* or *community situation.*

To understand where this emphasis on participation comes from, I looked widely at occupational therapy literature. The focus on participation has been encouraged since the First World War, when occupational therapy became a profession. As an example, Mary Reilly stated in a keynote lecture in 1962 that 'man, through the use of his hands as they are energized by mind and will, can influence the state of his own health' (p. 2). More recently, in her review of occupational therapy's epistemology, values, and relation to medicine, Yerxa (1992, p. 81) cites an 'optimistic view of people' as '*active*, capable, free, self-directed agents' versus medicine's view of people as '*passive*, incompetent, constrained, sick, controlled, pawns' [my emphasis]. Analysis of the reasoning behind occupational therapists' actions indicated they were constantly emplotting therapeutic encounters in which they recognize people with disabilities as active, holistic, knowing subjects (Mattingly, 1991).[3]

An interesting feature of occupational therapy discourse since the early 1980s has been the emphasis on *client-centred* practice (Department of National Health and Welfare and Canadian Association of Occupational Therapists, 1983, 1986, 1987; Canadian Association of Occupational Therapists [CAOT], 1991, 1997; Health Canada and Canadian Association of Occupational Therapists, 1993). Client-centred practice in occupational therapy is meant to enable participation so that people can realize their self-defined goals for a meaningful life. Concepts and categories in the 1983 Occupational Performance Model (refined in the 1997 Canadian Model of Occupational Performance) form the basis for a popular assessment procedure, the Canadian Occupational Performance Measure (COPM) (Law et al., 1990). The occupational therapist invites people to rate their satisfaction with their performance in any productive, leisure, or self-care occupations that are important to them in their environment. The COPM works by involving people in prioritizing and rating the importance of daily living, then rating their actual performance and level of satisfaction with those aspects of life. As assessment information is gathered, facts about people's daily lives are related to the occupational performance categories – defined as self-care, productivity, and leisure – that are depicted as occurring in an environment. Categories of performance and the environment are used to help people to understand, reflect on, and interpret their own participation. For instance, Petra later asked Carl: 'How are you doing in self-care? By self-care, I mean how often do you take a bath? Who does your laundry?' and 'Who gets you up in the morning?' She also encouraged him to analyse his environment by saying 'I am interested in knowing where you live and who you live with – generally how you live.'

Occupational therapy ideology assumes that people with mental health problems can be active participants in therapy and in their lives. For example, people are deliberately designated as active clients, consumers, or members, and the focus in assessment is to find out how people are participating in everyday life and in helping themselves. People like Carl are educated to think about their participation, and program facilities and schedules presume that people will participate. In fact the expenditures made in renovating hospital space or old houses give some degree of official recognition that people are expected to be active participants who are involved in helping themselves.

Concepts of participation are also present in the professional and governmental discourse of mental health services: participation is one of the key concepts in federal and provincial documents on mental health promotion; and the official brochures of mental health day programs portray people with mental health problems as participants in programs. These brochures have been developed by professionals, often with contributions from the people who attend the programs. For public relations purposes, the brochures are posted on bulletin boards or information racks in program facilities, and are used in public presentations such as mall displays during Mental Health Week. These materials are also used in the work of admission. They are circulated to agencies and professionals who might refer people to mental health day programs. In their discourse, such materials both recognize those who attend as active participants and define expectations that participation will occur. Segments from these descriptions state that the staff of these programs will:

... enable you to live a healthy, productive life. (Bayview)

... assist you in making any changes you wish to make in your life. (Clearcove)

... develop client's work skills (such as concentration, organization, responsibility) so as to train for job readiness. (Jackson Heights)

... teach you the skills needed to function effectively and develop environmental resources needed to support and strengthen your present level of functioning. (New Garden)

... help people learn to cope with life problems in a constructive manner. (Penrose)

... enhance your functioning in this community. (Rosehill)

Statements begin by indicating how staff will act, but they also describe people as active program participants who live in a 'community' with 'life problems' and 'environmental resources.' People are depicted as learners through references that staff will 'assist,' 'enable,' and 'teach,' and that participants will develop 'skills' and 'function.' Descriptions such as these suggest that staff play a catalyst, educator role while people are recognized as having the potential to be active, at least to the extent that they agree to participate in these programs. The public display of these materials presumes that people have the active power to read and learn about services on their own. Such documents also make a public statement that people who attend mental health day programs may have mental health problems but are not passive recipients of care. Instead, the descriptions recognize people as holistic, autonomous humans who ought to be invited, despite their problems, to participate in helping themselves.

It seems, then, that occupational therapists intend to promote empowerment: participation is invited in the design of facilities and schedules, in encounters with those who attend mental health day programs, and in public relations and admissions materials. In fact, occupational therapists are positive about working in these programs *because* of the emphasis on participation.

Objectifying Cases

If you continue to observe and listen to occupational therapists, you see that client participation is a veneer: clients rarely participate in the underlying organization of services. You can both see and feel the fundamental contradiction between espousing and encouraging participation in everyday situations, while at the same time defining people as psychiatric patients. How can such tension exist, with little professional awareness of the ways in which participation is undermined?

Each occupational therapist talked about practising 'in psychiatry,' defining occupational therapy with reference to this medical specialty. While the talk is about active clients and members, six of the seven occupational therapists (Neva was the exception) write about people as patients and categories of medical diagnosis. Official descriptions of people tend to begin something like 'This is a 38-year-old schizophrenic patient,' or program descriptions may identify the clientele as 'manic depressive patients.' Patients, by definition, are not active participants. Reliance on a patient discourse demonstrates the belief that people do not hold active power when it comes to their own health. Patients wait to be treated. They receive rather than participate in health services. Health professionals declare a moral responsibility to serve patients; in return, patients are responsible for presenting a body and mind to be acted on by professional experts.

Although a philosophical critique of passivity in a discourse about patients could be considerably expanded, an institutional ethnography aims to show the social organization of actual practices such as assessment. Here, the categorization of patients during assessment undermines participation by defining people as passive rather than active participants, by educating people to think of themselves as passive recipients of medical care, even when they are not being cared for by physicians.

Carol gives us an everyday example of the tension created by involving active participants while also categorizing them as patients:

I always work from the point of view that the patients know themselves best, better than I do, better than the psychiatrist does. Better than any of the other staff, they know what works for them, what's best for them ... it's not for me to say 'Oh, I think you can only work part-time – full time would be too much.' I ... just facilitate them looking at themselves.

Even when occupational therapists refer to people as clients or members in general discussion, in formal meetings they make references to patients. Almost without exception, people are described as patients in official health records. In hospital-based mental health day programs, virtually everyone, staff and people themselves, refer to patients. The concept of a patient has been generalized so much that the title of a book on feminist ethics and healthcare, *No Longer Patient* (Sherwin, 1992), jolts us into reflecting on societal assumptions that we will indeed be patient about waiting for someone else to make us healthy.

Assessment approaches also show how participation is contradicted and undermined. Rasha explains that she asks about people's typical days before they entered the program in order to find out:

what [a person's] life was like prior to the program and where we can see we might be able to make a difference.

While she is indicating the importance of people participating in assessment, she says 'where *we* can see *we* might be able to make a difference.' By using 'we,' is Rasha implying that it is now up to the expert occupational therapist to determine what is best? The program may or may not make a difference. If occupational therapists' concept of a person having active power is clear, might Rasha have said 'where we might guide a *person* to consider what changes *he or she* thinks are best'? The process of diagnostic categorization organizes power so that medical professionals are expected to care for passive patients. Rasha, like many others, perpetuates this organization of power by reproducing the categorization of patients in her everyday language.

References to patients and medical diagnostic categories seem inconsequential. After all, most people do not stay in mental health services forever. Besides, diagnostic categories are used to determine what treatment is appropriate. Can people not be active participants despite their labels? One problem is that labels stick. Although occupational therapists believe that people have active power, references to patients convey that, in a health context, people are passive patients. As well, people are stigmatized once they are categorized as psychiatric or mental patients. These stigmatizing categories educate people to think of themselves as disordered objects, such as schizophrenics or manic depressives, whose lives have been devalued by their mental state. They lose sight of their active potential to participate as worthy, holistic, autonomous agents who deserve equal opportunities to live. Instead of thinking how to participate in shaping their lives, people become preoccupied with their diagnosis, saying things like 'I think I've got to change my personality' (a person at Penrose). Or, as another person in a group with Rasha exclaimed one day:

I had a brainwave on the way over here today. What do you think of this? I think that I'm not really depressed. That diagnosis doesn't really fit. I think I'm actually hyper-stressed! (A person at Rosehill)

As we saw in the exchange between Petra and Carl, occupational therapists and others have an uphill struggle to encourage people in these programs to think of themselves as anything but passive medical objects. The message given is that patients have somehow lost their agency, their power, and their knowledge to decide what is best for themselves. Severe, diagnosed mental disorders *do* distort thinking and rob people of their power to understand themselves and the world. However, people retain some degree of active power to participate in and influence everyday life.

Beyond perpetuating ideas about passive patients in their speech, occupational therapists contribute directly to the categorization of patients. We previously saw Petra shifting Carl's attention from his psychiatric diagnosis to her categorization of everyday life. However, there are far more instances in which the process occurs in reverse. Information about active persons participating in everyday life is transformed into official categories that are used to monitor the mental status of mental patients and to organize mental health services. Here, the categories are diagnoses defined in the American Psychiatric Association's *Diagnostic and Statistical Manual of Mental Disorders (DSM).*[4] The transformation occurs during official discussions and in the documentation of occupational therapists' assessment information. Official discussions include intake meetings, assessment meetings, case coordination meetings, or rounds. At these official meetings, professionals discuss what they have learned about people before and after admission. While casual conversations include references to active clients and members, at official meetings, occupational therapists typically shift this information into the categories that guide psychiatrists in working with psychiatric patients. Carol's description to me shows how a psychiatric interpretation transforms information on participation into evidence of mental pathology:

ET   Daily schedule – what would you do with that? What would you be looking for?

Carol   I guess you can find out a lot of information by posing the question 'describe a typical day.' I use that a lot because I get a lot of information.

ET   What do you pick up – what kind of information?

Carol   What their level of activity is – if they're depressed, and if they're manic – if they're feeling abused, threatened – if they're compulsive housekeepers – that kind of thing – what their sleep patterns are –

that's important as well. And this gives you a really good idea of how they are functioning before [attending the program].

Sometimes the transformation is done by looking for medical behaviours like taking medication, as Rasha explains while looking at a weekly schedule sheet just completed by a woman who is very concerned about her medication:

Most people don't put in that they take their medication. So, in fact, this is very interesting to see, well number one, that she does take it as prescribed. But it seems to be a very important part of her life that she would even write it down on the page.

People are also transformed into patients in health records, starting with initial assessment and admission. Occupational therapy reports, like those used by other professions, are included as part of health records. These reports provide background or supporting information in the assessment of mental status. The importance of this information becomes clear when one realizes that the process of assessment is connected with the process of admission.

The assessment questions that Petra poses to Carl recognize people's subjective knowledge and autonomy to participate in shaping everyday life. In actual practice, occupational therapists, like other professionals, may conceptualize, categorize, and actually work with people as active persons. They assess whether people might benefit from admission to programs. As well, people often become involved in program activities long before the official diagnostic confirmation appears on a health record. Carol's and Rasha's comments above, however, show how occupational therapists use this information as a *medium*. In order to fit with official reporting and documentation processes, information about participation is interpreted as evidence of a person's mental health problem during assessment and admission.

Assessment and admission appear to be unbiased and objective processes in the scientific management of people with mental health problems. Yet these are not really objective because they operate with a specific but unstated ideology that the only diagnosis that counts is medical. Problems are located in individuals who need to submit to medical expertise for the purpose of psychiatric treatment. Mai describes some recent developments:

We have a new intake-discharge form – it's both things. And part of what we have to do on this is measure people's functioning. It's from the *DSM III-R*. We hadn't been using that but now we are. I find that it's an interesting way of looking at people. I always looked at people in that way, but now, it's an official thing that everybody has to do. So I don't know if other people find it more difficult or not. As an occupational therapist, you always look at the dysfunctional impairment and gauge where people are, and their abilities to function. Part of it is gauging their present functional level as you see them in the clinic, then comparing that against past function, the best they've done in the past year. So you're getting a picture of the possibilities for this person.

The process of psychiatric diagnosis seems to have improved, with its increasing emphasis on functional and social criteria, but the everyday process of categorizing people perpetuates the creation of patients who are dependent on professionals. The process is rein-forced each time selected facts about people's actual lives are col-lected by occupational therapists and other professionals. From the full narrative of people's lives in a social context, mental health pro-fessionals select only those facts that are relevant to diagnostic cate-gories of mental disorder in the *DSM*. Each diagnosis defines only a fragment rather than the full contextual experience of an active per-son. As well, the diagnosis individualizes the experience of mental disorder as if this is purely an individual, biological problem, despite the *DSM*'s inclusion of social and functional conditions. While a diagnosis guides professionals in treating people, acquisition of a *DSM* diagnosis invisibly buries their strengths and circumstances. People are transmuted from being active citizens into individualized, diagnostic categories – that is, into objects that, like mufflers in cars, need to be treated as faulty or deficient parts.

An interesting feature of medical categorization is that this social practice organizes power relations so that people are transformed into medical objects whether or not a physician is personally present. The problem or diagnosis must be entered on official records if a per-son is to qualify as a case for admission to mental health services. Then the diagnostic category is used to coordinate assessment infor-mation from various mental health professionals and to control pro-gram admission. As Britte says, in the absence of the psychiatrist, the practice is to 'make a little note to our medical director':

Whosever turn it is gets the chart as soon as possible, looks at the chart, interviews whoever made the referral, and, if they feel the patient is appropriate – or even if they don't actually – they make a little note to our medical director saying 'We feel this patient is appropriate or not' for whatever reasons – and he says what he thinks. So we review it, give our opinion, then the medical director looks at it. Generally, if we think they're appropriate, it's just a rubber stamp. We have rounds every Thursday afternoon, and if we disagree on whether a patient should be admitted or not, then we talk about it.

I emphasize that occupational therapists' contributions to assessment and admission are not controlled through face-to-face interaction with psychiatrists. Good psychiatrists draw people in as participants in assessing and helping to change their lives, and they value the diverse expertise of people whom they have diagnosed as having mental disorders. In part, the controlling power of psychiatric diagnosis is sustained by mental health professionals and those who use mental health services. In part, however, this controlling power is sustained by corporate interests in individualized, pharmaceutical treatments that require an individualized diagnosis of biological symptoms. Everyday interactions by occupational therapists, psychiatrists, and others differ from the institutional categorization and use of medical diagnoses. Acting together, assessment and admission transform active people into psychiatric‾patients and cases so completely that people refer to themselves as patients or cases even when they are no longer in a medical institution or undergoing medical treatment.

We will see in subsequent chapters that the process of objectification that transforms people into patients and cases has far-reaching ramifications if professionals are to enable people to become empowered, that is, to enable participation rather than caregiving. Action-oriented facilities and schedules and positive-sounding brochures make very little difference. All health professionals, whether or not they are medically oriented in their own work, are used as experts in gathering information on medical symptoms that determine access to health services. Other forms of health knowledge, such as occupational therapists' knowledge about enabling people to participate in solving daily living problems, are subordinated in the individualizing, objectifying processes of assessment and admission. Moreover, the definition of patients as objectified cases is the basis for individual case management, with its emphasis on individual rather than social action.

At the same time as it highlights participation, health professionals' literature refers to *patients*, as well as to *cases*, *case* studies, *case*loads, and numbers of *cases* studied. Yet cases are objects, not active participants who can be decision-making partners with professionals or otherwise involved in their own empowerment. As objects, cases are inert, unable to participate in the personal, social, and transformative learning process needed to change real-life situations. Change is limited because cases are protected from the risk taking that people face in their lives. Moreover, psychiatric cases continue to be stigmatized and segregated in society.

It is no wonder that those who invite participation in mental health day programs experience the tension of being different. They are simultaneously engaged in contradictory practices: as they contribute to the routines of assessment and admission, they are negating their good intentions of inviting people to participate. Instead of inviting participation, they are perpetuating the organization of caregiving, of individual, patient health *care*.

3

Individualizing Action

Empowerment is a process that invites participation in individual and collective actions, as well as in the organization of society. If we intend to enable others to become empowered, then we need to ask how invisible organizational processes determine possibilities for individual and collective action. One answer to this question has already been laid out: mental health services *individualize* action by assessing and admitting only *individual*, medically categorized patients. Mental health services have no cases that are not individuals: no group cases exist as in government departments of agriculture, which work not only with individual farmers but also with groups representing the collective interests of farmers. To see what happens to individual mental health cases, let us first look at how mental health professionals involve participants individually and collectively in day pro- grams, and then examine the routine organization of power in case management.

Facilitating Interdependence

There is an ongoing debate in the empowerment literature over the importance of collective versus individual action. The debate centres on differing views of autonomy and the potential for people to exert power alone or collectively. Broadly speaking, social analyses focus on collective action; psychological analyses focus on individual action. I have said that we participate in life by activating mind, body, and spirit. But I have also said that participation is shaped by the particular circumstances of our lives. The summary of empowerment offered in chapter 1 indicated that there are both individual and social elements. There is an interaction and interdependence between individual and collective action. The work of enabling empowerment, then, involves facilitating individuals to act both on their own and collectively.

Individualistic analyses are particularly helpful in understanding how mental, physical, spiritual, and other individual traits influence people's will and capacity for empowerment. An understanding of individuals is needed to learn how we participate in mind, body, and spirit in collective action. Social attitudes and practices may undermine empowerment if they stigmatize disability, aging, poverty, or other traits. But empowerment may be limited by individuals' personal sense of powerlessness, arising from a subdued will, lack of skill, or lack of technical support for engaging in the everyday world. Some people may believe that they ought to accept powerlessness as their natural condition.

Social analyses are also needed because they describe society, what some call the environment. Critical social analyses identify possibilities and barriers for social change, particularly the types of transformative change needed for empowerment. Social change occurs through collective action; and collective action occurs when people engage in consciousness raising, skill development, and spiritual transformation. Collective action enables individuals to act together in groups rather than individually. Collective action is needed to change the organization of power by state institutions, such as mental health services, but collective action depends on individuals participating. Conversely, participation in individual action that transforms experiences of power and the ability to exert power develops the foundation for collective action.

If we are to enable people to become empowered, we need to educate them to take individual action that enhances their personal feelings and thoughts of power and to feel and think like powerful persons. Where individuals seek spiritual transformation, we need to prompt them to see their own source of power in connection with a spiritual force beyond themselves.

Simultaneously, we need to facilitate individuals and groups to exert greater power through actions in everyday situations. To do this, we can coach them to develop skills, function, performance, and other behaviours that overtly demonstrate their power. For instance, one might facilitate some individual and collective action by coaching individuals to perform the instrumental functions required for everyday living. To become empowered, people need skills of some kind. Depending on their situations, people may need to look after themselves, organize attendants to look after them, find employment, manage money and shopping, organize transportation, decide health and social priorities, solve problems in everyday situations, participate in political actions, and serve on committees or other organizing bodies. It is crucial that we go beyond an instrumental view of life to ensure that people have the skills to take action in lobbying, activism, advocacy, community development, public education, and research.

The last two actions involve participants in another element in the empowerment process: the organization of society. On a local scale, one might educate individuals and groups to change the way power is exercised in friendships, in family and home circumstances, in employment, and in various community situations. These approaches develop natural forms of helping such as self-help and mutual aid, which strengthen social networks. On a broader scale, one might educate individuals and groups to develop philosophies, policies, procedures, financial resources, and legislation based on an ethical commitment to help those who are not yet empowered. Broad collective action is undertaken with awareness that historical practices of governing have resulted in some social groups (such as professionals) having control over others (such as patients).

In some instances, we might facilitate social change by acting *on behalf of* people. This makes sense for those in positions of authority where organizational processes, such as policies and legislation, can be written so that marginalized and powerful people become entitled to participate in defining how services will be organized and funded. While it is necessary to develop conditions that support rather than undermine empowerment, acting on behalf of people is not sufficient. A more direct approach is to facilitate collective action *with* people. As we examine individual and collective action in occupational therapy, we can see how the transformation of feelings, thoughts, actions, and organization are interconnected.

Facilitating Individual and Collective Action

As I became familiar with the design of day program facilities and the processes of assessment and admission, I was also observing and asking what occupational therapists do with people each day. In our discussions, each occupational therapist talked a lot about working with individuals, while emphasizing their involvement with community groups and services. They told me that they went beyond official expectations for working with individuals in hospitals, for instance, in exploring 'the person–environment fit':

I hope I'm not giving the impression that I think that it's strictly individual – because you have to understand the whole environment. That's a key of occupational therapy – the environment, the person–environment fit, the whole social milieu – understanding its impact and that it isn't always the person.

Neva describes her involvement in social action in terms of 'working with [the environment].' She is particularly interested in making clear her recognition that 'it isn't always the person.'

A commitment to change the environment seems to be accompanied by facilitating some people to engage in local collective action. Every program includes sessions in which people engage in the social action of planning the day and future events. Planning emphasizes the overall program rather than individual actions. Sometimes these sessions are called Morning Meeting, Warm-Up Group, Check-In Meeting, or Weekly Planning Meeting. In these contexts, planning involves daily or weekly activities; there may also be talk about barriers and ideas for changing transportation, sheltered employment, or subsidized housing. As these topics arise, people describe problems or solutions associated with using buses or finding places to work and live. Sometimes people get together to send a letter; join a local march; call politicians and managers to get information; negotiate with hospital managers for patient rights and privileges; write proposals to get funding for recreation, employment, or housing; or otherwise engage in collective action.

Neva says that a large amount of her work involves program members in community issues. She has people write briefs, prepare speeches for community events, and develop public relations materials. As well, Neva is engaged in developing transitional employment options that support people in real employment situations. When I asked Mai about social action, she immediately replied:

One of the first things I got involved in [was] the transition house association. I got asked to help – it was initially just a general meeting of anyone in the community interested in getting something organized that was going to be a help to victims of violence. Specifically, we were talking about women and children. And, there was already an idea to have a shelter. That had been discussed before – so that was their main focus. So I got involved in that at a general meeting. Then I joined the board. Then I was on the board of directors for a couple of years. And since then, I've been involved with them from time to time, certainly as a referral source. And also, at times, doing sessions, seminars with some of the women.

In another example, Petra describes her involvement in developing a new group home:

I meet with them once a week. And what I do with them has really varied. When all three of them were new to the house, I spent a lot of time doing meal preparation and budgeting; we did up a household cleaning schedule, those kinds of things. And over the last couple of months, there's been a lot of interpersonal problems and I've gone in there and we've basically had a group therapy session for an hour with all of them. I mean their concerns, gripes, and calling each other names.

Working on behalf of people, the occupational therapists all reported that they are members of committees, groups, volunteer boards of directors, and various organizations advocating for and participating in the development of transportation, housing, employment, recreation, and other aspects of community life. Britte and Rasha listed social action as part of their work in developing special YMCA programs for people who live in the community and who have been diagnosed with a mental disorder. Britte was assisting with the development of a sheltered workshop for mentally handicapped people and an extended care nursing home for people with mental handicaps; Carol was participating on various community committees and a task force examining the reorganization of provincial mental health services. In exploring social action with Jill, I asked:

ET Is it fair to say that your advocacy is primarily with the individual, and that you're not really involved in broader social action?

Jill No – both. I was quite active in this Employment Incentive Committee a couple of years ago. And that was a bunch of us – all the organizations from the community ... as well as people from the hospital. And we were lobbying the government to change that whole system ... the occupational therapy director is very supportive of us – always wanting an occupational therapist to be on these community-based committees – so that we can give our input. I think there are a number of other committees. But that is the one that I was involved with. And the housing program that I'm involved in. I have a lot of say in that. That's all community-based.

When I followed up by asking how people were involved in the Employment Incentive Committee, she replied:

That's a fairly political group – and a lot of that was based on client comments and case histories from clients. So that was the way they were involved.

As I reflected on occupational therapists' involvement in social action on behalf of, and with people, I realized that there is some official expectation for occupational therapists to make collective, social action part of everyday practice: program facilities (space) and schedules (time) are structured to make both individual and collective action possible.

The group rooms provide recognition that collective action is expected to occur at least within programs. Office space for meeting with individuals is equalled or surpassed by space for working collectively with people. Each program includes at least one room called a Group Room with chairs and sofas arranged in a circle, often with a flip chart or blackboard at hand. As well, the kitchen, workshop, and general work rooms are used with groups and individuals. All programs have some type of lounge in which people meet collectively without professionals during coffee breaks and between scheduled activities. Overall, it seems that facilities have been designed for collective as well as individual action.

In addition, time is routinely scheduled for collective as well as individual action. The typical day includes individual time and at least two types of group events. My estimate, from analysing schedules and observing over a number of weeks, is that occupational therapists spend at least 35 per cent of their time working with people collectively, equal to the 35 per cent of time spent with individuals and their immediate social contact persons (family, social workers, etc.). As well, 10 per cent of time (sometimes more, or none, in any week) is spent in local or broad collective action, with and sometimes on behalf of people. The other 20 per cent of occupational therapists' time is spent in meetings and documentation that may organize possibilities for integrating individual and collective action.

More organizational support appears to exist in position descriptions, which indirectly include collective and individual action. Rasha's 'Position Description' (figure 3.1) lists a typical array of duties.

Of particular interest in figure 3.1 are the two statements that I have highlighted in bold. The statement 'implement appropriate treatment programs using dyadic or group intervention' encourages occupational therapists to work collectively with groups, and not to confine contact to individuals; the statement 'participate in determining the philosophy, objectives, and policies of the department' supports professional involvement in shaping organizational processes. Both statements in this Position Description offer an official window of opportunity for occupational therapists to involve people in developing some aspects of the program philosophy, objectives, and policies, in social as well as individual action.

The Canadian Workload Measurement System: Occupational Therapists (WMS) also encourages occupational therapists to engage in collective as well as individual action. The system documents time spent in working with individuals: 'direct patient care' and 'indirect patient care' are documented in five-minute time units (note that a patient discourse threads through many occupational therapy documents and statements). Units are attributed to individuals on time unit records, even if people are engaged collectively in various sizes of groups. However, one section of 'non–patient care activities' (i.e., time *not* allocated to individuals) lists 'service to community,' including 'board/community function,' 'public education,' 'consultation,' and 'service to profession.' Where people are involved in collective action, the time for this type of practice can be recorded.[1]

As anyone who has observed occupational therapists knows, everyday practice is highly individualized. Nevertheless, occupational therapists' commitment to and involvement in collective action is important to highlight. If one observes occupational thera-

FIGURE 3.1
Occupational Therapist: Position Description (Rosehill)*

List of Duties:

Upon referral the occupational therapist shall:

- evaluate the patient's condition and level of function, through the use of interview, observation, or assessment
- determine treatment goals, discussing these with the patient and informing him or her of the nature and risks of treatment
- *implement appropriate treatment programs using dyadic or group intervention*
- progress, adjust, and terminate programs ensuring appropriate referral and follow-up where indicated
- assess the effectiveness of treatment programs
- refer patient to other therapeutic services in the department, hospital, or community
- record method and results of evaluation; program goals and outcome; disposition of the patient
- contribute to the clinical team by participating in the process of diagnosis, goal development, and patient management, and giving clinical observations

The occupational therapist shall also:

- *participate in determining the philosophy, objectives, and policies of the department*
- participate in the evaluation of own performance and that of others under his or her direction
- participate in and contribute to programs of staff education and orientation
- maintain necessary records, reports, and statistical data
- supervise auxiliary staff or students as directed
- promote and practise good interpersonal and interdepartmental relationships
- assist in the administration of the department when requested
- make effective use of supplies, equipment, and facilities
- assist with all departmental programs as directed
- perform other related duties

*Sample of official Position Description, Rosehill

pists fully, as I did, and looks at this profession's literature, one finds examples of occupational therapists agitating for change in homes, schools, workplaces, training centres, in shopping and banking, transportation, communication, and virtually every other area of daily life. The occupational therapists studied here were members of boards of directors, government committees, management planning groups, lobby groups, and legislative groups, working on behalf of and sometimes with people with mental health problems. Important to highlight is the fact that occupational therapists tend to be involved in collective action outside paid work time.

Individualizing Case Management

While learning about possibilities for facilitating individual and collective action, I began to see that this feature, too, is part of the disjuncture, the tension between enabling participation and caregiving. Mental health professionals such as occupational therapists facilitate a range of actions that seem consistent with enabling empowerment, yet this work occurs with individually diagnosed patients. How can this contradiction persist in the same time and place with the same people?

I began to see how this part of the tension works in daily practice when I asked occupational therapists about social action. Jill did not point to her focus on individual action but, rather, talked about trying to 'do it all' while handling a caseload of 80 individuals in the past, now only '40 people':

It's crazy – I used to have 80 people on my caseload before the other therapist came. Now we still carry about 40 people each and that's too much – I used to be taking work home and doing it at 1 in the morning. There are so few community resources here that you have to keep working away and getting involved in far more than in some other communities.

Jill refers to her attempts to expand the 'few community resources' by 'working away and getting involved.' She perceives that she has too much to do without noting that she is putting a huge amount of time and energy into managing individuals. Her strong emphasis on individual action is taken for granted, while social action is assumed to be a peripheral part of practice that is squeezed into her work with individuals.

The emphasis on individuals is not surprising if you read about occupational therapy's conceptual models, for instance, Canada's evolving Model of Occupational Performance (Department of National Health and Welfare & Canadian Association of Occupational Therapists, 1983; Canadian Association of Occupational Therapists, 1997). This model focuses on individual performance, even though there is recognition that individual action is shaped by an environment. Concepts of occupational performance have a strong grounding in the individualistically oriented theories of human development of Maslow, Piaget, and others. A huge proportion of occupational therapy literature describes programs designed to enable individuals to enhance components of performance that have been lost or never developed, and research referring to mental health is predominantly directed at individuals' cognitive and emotional growth.

Moreover, individualism runs through occupational therapy discourse, particularly in the concept of independence. Talk about social action is overshadowed by program mission statements that emphasize individual responsibility. Besides, everyday practice is individualized by the processes of individual goal setting and individual case coordination. These organizational processes form the basis for documenting individual cases and evaluating the quality and quantity (efficiency) of individual case management.

Carol's talk displays occupational therapy discourse on individual *independence*:

Enabling independence is the core of what I try to do. I can't give someone independence, nor can anyone else. But you try to give the person the tools so that they can be as independent as they can. Now, how do I do that? I guess through teaching of skills, helping them to problem solve, helping them to identify, first of all what the problem is. Then doing some priority setting and some goal planning. Re-evaluating, coming back – alright, did this work? Maybe it didn't. Let's try something else. How do you feel about this today? Not so good. OK, let's look at this another way. And, I always come back to – it's your goals – the patient's goals. OK, then, 'enabling independence.' How would I actually do the enablement? I guess, start at the beginning with the assessment or with the work that I've done with the client. Find out what their goal is. What priority they put on their goal. OK, let's look at how we can work on the first goal, second goal, and so on. Then we help them to arrive at how they are going to approach that particular goal. For example, if they're looking at job skills, you might do a vocational history. You look at what kind of things they've worked at. What kinds of work would they like to do? Often, an issue is how much can they work? If they haven't been very well, and they're still a little fragile, I might help them to look at working part-time instead of full-time to start.

Carol links independence to individual 'skills' and the ability to 'problem-solve.' Skills and problem-solving ability are presented as the 'tools' of independence. The actual practice of 'enabling independence' is to engage an individual in 'assessment' to find out 'what their goal is' and 'what priority they put on their goal.'

The emphasis on individual action is also promoted by official statements about individual responsibility. As Britte talks about the mission and philosophy of Bayview day program, we can see how the overwhelming focus on individual action is rooted in documents that hold people individually responsible for improving their mental health:

In our mission statement and goals and objectives, we specify that we're trying to help people take responsibility for their illness and care. Our whole philosophy attempts to attack the belief that people are controlled by their illness. From day one, we ask people to set goals for change, to say 'this is what I'm going to do to help myself get better.' One lady this morning talked about 'getting the crawlies.' She has come quite a way in accepting responsibility for her illness. There was a time when she would not accept the fact that she could do anything about it. And she still says that there are bad days when she can't do anything about it. But now, she will take steps like going out and calling someone up. It's a hard row to hoe. Changing – helping a person change their beliefs. You can't change it for them. A lot of our educational programming looks at that – at ways to change behaviour. And you can't change behaviour without changing the beliefs that lead to that behaviour.

Britte reiterates the institutional position that individual people 'take responsibility for their illness and care.' The mission is to help people to accept and act on that individual responsibility by 'helping a person change their beliefs' and their 'behaviour.' The program mission makes no reference to facilitating collective action, assisting the community to develop support services, or changing funding policies to provide part-time employment and social support. Yet such action might help people who are 'getting the crawlies' to 'take steps like going out and calling someone up.'

Carol's discussion of independence and responsibility also refers to goal-setting and case coordination. Assessing individuals and finding out 'what their goal is' and 'what priority they put on their goal' are cornerstone processes in individual case management. Carol indicates that the goal-setting process is one of determining a 'first goal' then a 'second goal.' The actual management of goals is achieved by asking people 'how they are going to approach that particular goal.'

The individualization of these goals becomes clearer when she talks about helping people to think about performance, or 'skills.' Individual skill development is a strategy for facilitating action such as 'working part-time instead of full-time to start.' Given the difficulties that people with mental health problems have with skill development and planning, this work is important. Particularly when mental difficulties last for more than a few months, individuals do have problems that require them to develop basic skills for living in society.

Rasha discusses individual responsibility in relation to her work of managing cases such as Brenda:

I guess it's a matter of letting them make their own decisions. Helping them deal with the consequences. Realizing that they are responsible for whatever happens to them. Now obviously, some people have chemical imbalances and so on. But they can also have at least some control over whether they take their medications, or seek help when they need it. We help them to realize that they have a right to feel what they feel and that they have the right to make their own choices, and the ability to do so. But oftentimes, it takes time guiding them through those choices, and guiding them through the consequences, and guiding them to decide what they want to do next.

We warn them that 'we can teach you to set some goals and learn some techniques to manage whatever stresses are in your life ... It's not going to be easy. Staff will be tough with you. If you say you're going to do certain goals, we'll ask you if you did them and why not if you didn't. But we're also understanding. We're here because we know that people get over their head and need help getting organized and getting to know themselves. But if you're willing to work at it, you can make some changes in your life. These won't be changes we come up with. They will be changes you say you want to make your life better in your view. It's whatever you want to do. You won't make all the changes in your life in the program. But we'll help you get started.'

Whereas Carol gives examples of individual case management, Rasha describes how case management actually works. Based on individualistic ideas of independence and responsibility, case management monitors individual action in which people take responsibility for managing their own lives. It is sometimes taken for granted that individuals' problems arise from their lack of organization, self-knowledge, and mental pathology. Rasha implies that individuals like Brenda have mental difficulties primarily because they are faulty managers who have little self-awareness. While this may be partly true, an individualized approach negates social conditions that we know trigger mental health problems or make them worse.

Another implication is that the onus is on individuals to solve their personal problems. As Rasha states, 'goals' are the mechanism for exercising responsibility and making choices. Her job is to 'teach you to set some goals and learn some techniques to manage whatever stresses are in your life.' While Rasha's job is to 'help you get started,' she warns that 'you won't make all the changes in your life in the program.' She assures Brenda, however, that 'we never just drop people on their own.' We learn that Rasha understands that it is 'not going to be easy' for Brenda, since staff like Rasha will 'be tough with you.' Rasha holds Brenda individually responsible for meeting her goals by asking her if she met them and to give reasons if she did not. To soften the tone of vigilance, Rasha empathizes with Brenda. She says 'we know that people get over their head and need help getting organized and getting to know themselves.' Rasha makes sure she injects the whole process with a tone of enthusiasm and hope. With overtones of a work ethic, Rasha promises that if she is 'willing to work at it,' Brenda can, as an individual, 'make some changes' in her life. The belief in Brenda's active power and personal responsibility as an individual is consistent with the individual elements of empowerment. Yet these kinds of statements offer no recognition that Brenda's empowerment requires collective as well as individual action.

Case management is not listed as such on program schedules. Nevertheless, individual case management is pervasive and reduces possibilities for facilitating collective action. Case management begins with assessment and admission and consists of various interconnecting processes so that even collective group sessions are actually attending to individual goals. Now you can see that assessment and admission are not discrete. They are interconnected, foundational processes for individual goal setting and case coordination. Individualized goals guide decision making, program involvement, and the overall orientation to change. In the end, progress on individual goals determines discharge and follow-up from mental health services.

To illustrate, Rasha reminds Brenda of her individual responsibility. She then explains the purpose of a goal-setting group:

FIGURE 3.2
Goal Setting: Brenda's Weekly Goals (Rosehill)*

Week 1:	Week 3:
1 Make bed daily	1 Read 1 chapter nightly
2 Do dishes nightly	2 Make bed each morning
3 Do some laundry over weekend	3 Make 3 positive statements daily
4 One compliment to family	4 Organize spare room Thursday and Friday
	5 Go to doctor's appointment on Wednesday
Week 2:	6 Go swimming Wednesday
1 Do laundry on Tuesday	7 Organize bedroom and kitchen
2 Bathe animal on Monday	8 Cut friend's hair
3 Wednesday – visit from social worker	9 Visit Manpower and check paper daily
4 Go to aquacize Wednesday	10 Follow diet
5 Thursday, organize 1 closet	
6 Friday – organize 2nd closet	
7 Do dishes nightly	
8 Make bed each morning	

*List produced during goal-setting group

We help you set goals for yourself and then it's up to you to complete those goals. They aren't our goals for you – they are goals you set for yourself. We also help you to set goals which are suitable to your situation since our focus is on helping you to cope with your life outside here – your work and the people in your life ... so you work with other people in the group. But you all may have different goals. There's a goal-setting group where you figure out your goals for each week and report back to the group on the goals from the week before.

Figure 3.2 provides a sample of the individual action that Brenda identified through goal setting over three successive weeks. Brenda's goals were generated by asking her, in turn, to list goals while other group members listened and contributed ideas. Each group member did the same thing while a team member recorded what was said. The list consists of goals for Brenda's individual action. There is no comparable list of goals that would engage Brenda in collective action.

These individual goals form the framework for program sessions that serve as a mechanism for case coordination. To illustrate, figure 3.3 lists Brenda's 'assertiveness goals' over the same three weeks as the goals listed in figure 3.2. Brenda's goals for individual action are addressed by developing assertiveness goals described as 'give one

FIGURE 3.3
Case Coordination: Brenda's Assertiveness Goals (Rosehill)*

	Homework Review	Assertive Area of Concentration	Homework Assigned
Week 1	new to group	compliments to family	give 1 compliment per day to anyone
Week 2	make compliments	positive statements	think and express positive feelings
Week 3	3 positive statements	receiving negative feedback	write 3 positive things per day; think before reacting

*List produced during assertiveness group

compliment per day to anyone' or 'write three positive things per day.'

These diverse actions may be discussed informally, such as Rasha asking Brenda in the hall or over coffee how she was doing in getting to swimming or following her diet. Alternatively, goals may be reviewed formally, usually in individual or group sessions, which provide professionals with information to be inserted in individual health records under the heading of 'Progress.' Furthermore, Rasha formally reported Brenda's progress at *case coordination* meetings, where occupational therapists and other professionals report to each other on progress related to individual goals. Generally, case coordination meetings are linked with *rounds*. Rounds are the most official of these meetings, typically chaired by the team psychiatrist, who facilitates discussion by the professional team on individual cases.

Individualization becomes even more apparent when one traces everyday practice to the documentation used to account for the quality and efficiency of practice. It is in documents that *individual case management* is most visible. Mental health professionals are primarily accountable for the quality and efficiency of individual case management. An extended section of Rasha's job description (figure 3.4) shows that her work is described as 'case coordination' as well as occupational therapy. Rasha's time is recorded in five-minute units as individual 'patient' time and community time. While occupational therapy's Workload Management System (WMS) reports social action under a category of time for 'community service activities,' WMS data, for the most part, are used internally in occupational therapy staffing decisions.

FIGURE 3.4
Occupational Therapist: Position Description (Rosehill)*

Case Coordinator
Roles and Responsibilities

The 'Case Coordinator' is responsible for coordinating all aspects of the care of the patient, under the direction of the Program Director, and is also responsible for discipline-specific activities for the program. He/she consults with all members of the multidisciplinary team to effectively use each member's expertise in the planning and delivery of care.

SPECIFICALLY THE CASE CO-ORDINATOR WILL:

Assessment
1 Ensure availability of relevant data from the patient, family, and significant others, and from previous records
2 Collaborate with the patient, team members, and significant others in order to establish priorities of care and to identify problems on an ongoing basis
3 Complete an initial clinical note within seven working days of admission

Patient Care Planning
1 Ensure the development of a treatment plan with realistic goals in consultation with the multidisciplinary team
2 Interpret the treatment plan to the patient and seek the patient's willingness to proceed with it

Implementation of Treatment Plan
1 Coordinate the implementation of the treatment plan
2 Review, evaluate, and revise the treatment plan on an ongoing basis
3 Document the minimum of one weekly progress note using a goal-oriented format

Discharge Planning
1 Commence discharge planning from the day of admission to ensure the patient is adequately prepared
2 Ensure completion of all necessary discharge documentation by appropriate professionals
3 Complete the Case Coordinator's portion of the discharge summary within three working days of discharge

*Sample of Position Description at Rosehill

Occupational therapy is made officially accountable for the *quality* of practice through the use of documentary processes called quality assurance.[2] Occupational therapists, like other mental health professionals, are accountable for the quality of individual case management. As Neva says:

Quality assurance, and all those notions ... they're very valid and they're good. But at the same time, they lead you to develop really structured programs, with very clear objectives and goals, so that you can then say that your client is meeting the objectives and goals.

In our introduction to Neva in chapter 1, we heard that one source of tension for her is around documentation ('hospital quality assurance and program kinds of stuff ... charting, statistics'), which 'keeps you quite attached to the medical model although you're trying to work with something that's very different.'

Health services management has instituted a large array of documentary mechanisms for controlling quality. Mental health day programs operate with only a few of those used in other hospital-funded services. Two of the main documentary mechanisms for managing quality here are the health record and the health record audit instrument.

The health record[3] is the central document in the management of quality. All health records are individualized. There are no records that carry equal weight in accounting for professional facilitation of collective action. The full health record includes documentation of the individual case: admission/entry, consent, referral (registration), background information ('history'), prior admissions, medical assessment (history, current status), assessment data from other professionals on the team, medical orders, 'patient' goals, progress (completed by all ongoing services) related to individual goals, other letters and reports (e.g., lab and consultant reports), discharge (referral to others, medical report), and other documentation related to a case.

Rasha describes the everyday process of documenting case management in a health record:

You write the problem list. Then you link that to the goal sheet. Then you link that to the progress notes. In the progress notes, I try to mention the problems, like Brenda's finances, and refer to them by the number from the problem sheet. But the progress note is more often a narrative description of what's going on with the person right now – symptoms, mood, that kind of thing – as well as the instrumental behaviours that the goals are linked to.

Individual action is based on a documented 'problem list' of individual problems. Individual problems are translated onto a 'goal

FIGURE 3.5
Categories for Auditing Health Records (Occupational Therapy) (Rosehill)*

Identification

Referral

Time Reference

Evaluation Methods

Intervention Plan

Discharge Summary

Frequency of Documentation

Signature

Corrections

*Extracted from health records, Rosehill

sheet' of individual goals. Work done in relation to individual goals is recorded in 'progress notes.' It is Rasha's documentation of individual problems, goals, and progress that is reviewed for quality assurance. As she says:

If I was doing strictly OT [occupational therapy] and not the case coordination part, it would be much easier for me to describe a meal assessment in detail. I could describe how they measured, or whether they could measure. Whereas with case coordination, when you're dealing with so many other issues that aren't necessarily occupational therapy–related, I just couldn't see myself putting in the time, the energy, or even feeling that it's that important to put all that detail down in a note. For instance, if he had difficulty measuring, I might put down 'had difficulty with measuring, will buy measures' or something, and go on from there rather than describing the whole thing. Reporting details about a meal assessment is very much constrained by the fact that I case coordinate, and I have to deal with medication issues, and marital issues and so on, which all come up.

The related health record audit instrument works in tandem with the health record in monitoring the quality of case management.

FIGURE 3.6
Caseload and Service Time per Case: Management Information System (MIS) Primary
Data Categories (Rosehill)

New referrals (source date of admission)
No shows (source: time data)
Missed visits (source: time data)
Length of stay in working days (source: discharge date less admission date)
Average daily attendance (source: time data/sometimes kept as a separate, aggregate
   program data form – group attendance)
Number of visits of 3 hours or less (source: time)
Number of visits of more than 3 hours (source: time)
Closed files (source: cases with termination dates in that month)

Additional categories (New Garden MIS):
Number of patients at end of previous month
Number of patients at end of the month

Information in a health record both organizes and is fitted to the categories on the typical audit form (see figure 3.5). The audit manages the quality of practice by reviewing the documented evidence of individual action. The review examines whether an individual referral has been authorized, services have been dated, and assessments ('evaluation methods') have identified 'strengths and deficits' and 'goals' for case coordination. The 'intervention plan' is evidence of 'individual/group' practice based on individual goals.

Occupational therapy is also accountable for the *quantity* of practice. Quantity is judged by the efficiency of handling individual cases. Efficiency is a textual object that is calculated as a measure of the number of cases managed over time. Data on time are entered in a Workload Management System (WMS), whereas data on cases are entered in a Management Information System (MIS) compatible with provincial and federal data requirements. An MIS sets out informational requirements by defining the facts required for the management of an institution. Typically, an MIS records the numbers of cases served, and the numbers of visits or services provided per case (see figure 3.6). In mental health services, caseloads are measured by aggregating the number of days of attendance of all cases of individuals and the number of individual cases discharged from the system each month. The MIS makes the everyday practice of all staff, including occupational therapists, accountable for the number of individual cases managed, their 'length of stay' (in days), and their frequency of contact (number of 'visits'). By calculating the number of cases handled per month, the MIS also provides an aggregate calculation of the efficiency of managing multiple individual cases (i.e., 'caseloads') by the mental health team as a whole. When one is attempting to facilitate collective as well as individual action – to engage in social action on the side as it were – one experiences the pressure Jill described earlier in keeping track of a 'caseload' of over 80 individuals.

For professionals such as occupational therapists, the MIS, and to some extent the WMS, set productivity expectations. In essence, data requirements for the MIS and WMS determine how occupational therapists and other team members spend their day. Although there are variations among team members, occupational therapists experience implicit pressure to carry caseloads that are similar to those of other professionals. In other words, the MIS and WMS standardize professional practice so that the individualized management of psychiatric cases is emphasized regardless of a profession's interest in facilitating collective action toward social change. MIS and WMS data requirements ensure that the majority of the day will be spent in facilitating individual action.

I do not negate the importance of individuals or individual action. As a philosophy, individualism urges us to recognize individuals as active participants with some degree of autonomy, active power, and ability to take responsibility for their actions. This type of analysis shows how individualism works in individual case management. Facts about individuals are managed as a way of coordinating and controlling the many health practices that comprise mental health services. In managing individual cases, professionals actively participate with each other, with managers, and with individual patients in what Dorothy Smith calls an *ideological circle* (1987, 1990a). This refers to a textual practice in which facts are extracted from real experience then used to explain and organize that experience. People's lived experience and the context of that experience are represented by individual diagnoses – that is, the complexity of people's lives is translated into categories of diagnosis so that patients/cases can be managed individually. Consequently, individual cases are coached to identify individual goals relevant to the mental facts of their diagnoses. Case coordination may facilitate collective and individual action, but all action is related to individual goals. The completion of case coordination (i.e., program discharge) is then based on progress relevant to individualized goals.

Documented problems, goals, and progress in case coordination provide the facts required to manage *quality assurance* in practice; numbers of diagnostic cases provide the facts required to manage *efficiency* in dealing with the quantity of cases admitted. Quality assurance and efficiency are not real; rather, they are concepts, created as textual objects that appear to be objective and neutral. On the contrary, these concepts are subjective, biased, and ideological. In mental health services, quality assurance and efficiency use only those facts that are relevant to individual cases and their psychiatric diagnoses. Even when collective action is part of practice, these facts make mental health professionals accountable primarily for facilitating individual action.

Collective action is encouraged in everyday practice, but professionals cannot count this as real work. Individual case management is so firmly embedded in the organizational framework of mental health services that collective action is officially and statistically irrelevant as a mental health practice. Individual medical diagnoses are not merely a guide for treatment; they are used to organize health services to be individualized and medically oriented. In essence, the work of managing individual cases is all that literally *counts*.

4

Controlling Collaboration

Empowerment is a process of participating in individual and collective action so that power and resources can be shared equitably. Power is shared through *collaboration*, the process of working with others in interdependent relations characterized by reciprocity and mutuality: giving and taking, helping and receiving help. The interdependence of collaboration makes this a horizontal rather than a hierarchical relation.

Identification of this third feature shows the complexity of empowerment: participation is important, but it needs to extend into collective as well as individual action; moreover, participation needs to occur in collaboration with others, rather than under their direction. We already know how psychiatric categorization creates individually diagnosed patients who are officially known only as passive objects of caregiving, even if they participate in the everyday processes of case management. We will now look at the opportunities for sharing power in everyday practice, tracing these to processes of decision making.

Encouraging Collaborative Decision Making

Decision making is both a skill and a highly contextual negotiation over the division of power. When we make decisions we are asking, Who will do what, under what circumstances? Who is responsible for what? What are the possible consequences? Who can be trusted to follow decisions? Under what circumstances might decisions be changed? Decision making that is collaborative includes: clarification of diverse assumptions and beliefs of all persons connected with a decision; analysis of a situation from each partner's perspective (analysis of strengths as well as problems); identification of possible sequences for action from each partner's perspective; negotiation to identify the practical implications of each action and the potential of each action for enhancing the empowerment of everyone involved; negotiation to decide the method of selecting action (majority vote, rotating roster, delphi method, random draw); reflection to ensure that power has been shared equally in the decision-making process; selection of action; and evaluation of the equality of decision-making power after action has been taken.

Collaborative decision making generally involves a dramatic change for both professionals and those with whom we work. Beliefs and assumptions that underpin decision making need to shift so that we move away from the traditional hierarchical organization of decision making by professionals towards reciprocity, mutuality, symmetry, partnership, and other collaborative, horizontal forms of relating that are fundamental to empowerment. To make this shift, professionals and those who use our services need to adopt a new ethic for decision making: that we are all responsible for creating equitable opportunities for everyone to participate in decision making.

The implication of this ethical commitment for professionals is that we must dismantle the unequal *banking* concept (a term coined by Freire and others) that professionals are the only people who can put expertise 'in the bank,' so to speak. Traditionally, professionals and others have assumed that everyone else draws professional expertise and knowledge from banks of professional knowledge. Collaborative decision making operates as a cooperative, not a bank. Using a cooperative model, professionals and others would voice their own perspectives and listen to alternate perspectives. Although their contributions would differ, they would accord equal value to one another's work and ideas in negotiating decisions, each one contributing to the best of her or his ability. To embed collaboration in institutions, policies, funding, legislation, and other official documents would entitle all parties to have equal opportunities for voicing their views and making the decisions that govern what can be done. In this way, collaboration would be routinely organized as an everyday practice.

Collaborating in Everyday Practice

Collaborative decision making was a common feature of the day programs I observed. Rather than tell people what is best for them, professionals repeatedly encouraged them to make decisions in at least five areas: program participation, personal goals, individual case coordination, personal preferences in the weekly program structure, and program evaluation. A brief look at each of these shows how collaboration actually occurs in mental health services.

Program participation may be undermined officially by categorizing people as patients and cases, and limited by the official practice of individual case management, but collaboration is evident in the everyday discussions, work, and planning that characterize program participation. Although many day programs are in hospital-based settings, people decide whether or not to attend each day, in contrast to attending treatment sessions on doctors' orders. In the various activities scheduled throughout the day, people decide whether or not to participate without any direct financial incentive. Moreover, people know what is happening and can decide what to attend since they generally receive a copy of the weekly schedule on admission and can always refer to a copy that is posted on a large schedule board in the lounge or main hall. People are free to decide how much, how, when, and with whom they participate. In collaboration with mental health professionals, they decide whether or not to participate in assertiveness, stress management, time management, goal-setting, weekly or weekend planning, food services, maintenance, clerical work, industrial subcontracting, and other sessions. There is no doubt that professional referrals (particularly from The Doctor) may be taken as an order rather than as choice. But, as Petra tells Mike, a person who is thinking about participating in a mental health program,

Would it help if I gave you a bit of information on the program and how it works? Then maybe you can decide from there whether you want to take part.

The decision is ultimately Mike's. Every occupational therapist I observed frequently used the phrase 'you can decide.' People were reminded over and over that they have choice and control with regard to their decision to participate in programs.

Collaborative decision making is also evident when people set personal goals. It sounds contradictory to say that managed cases actively share power in decision making, yet, in the last chapter, Rasha was shown prompting Brenda to make her own decisions

about goals and to incorporate these into assertiveness goals. Now
we can hear Britte referring to decisions about goals when she says
'We ask people to set goals for change ... you can't change it for
them.'

And as Rasha says:

I guess it's a matter of letting them make their own decisions. Helping them
deal with the consequences. Realizing that they are responsible for whatever
happens to them.

Rasha's use of the word 'letting' suggests that it is actually the professional who controls people's opportunities to make decisions. But
even the intention of relinquishing control is not a characteristic of
traditionally dominant professionals.

I also heard occupational therapists advocating for people to be
partners in the decision making associated with individual case coordination. Jill stresses people's ability to know what is best. She
describes occupational therapists as 'spokesmen'[1] for people in team
meetings that otherwise exclude them from decision making:

We often act as spokesmen for the individual. I know I have in the past. If so
and so would like to live independently – or in supportive housing. Sometimes the majority of people on the team are not looking at the desires of the
client. And we're often the spokesmen there saying 'but this is what they
want to do.' Or work is a good example. We had a real row here a while ago.
Some social centre in the community was hiring on some people. They had a
grant and were hiring on people. So a lot of people wanted their clients to go
and work there. And some of the clients weren't interested. So it was other
people deciding what's best for the client. So often times, we're the ones who
have to sit with the team and say 'but this person doesn't want ...' So we try
to facilitate that – that it's the individual's life and they want to make
these decisions – and don't you think we have to respect that? Sometimes it
works – not all the time.

Jill is not going so far as to suggest that decision making needs to
be an equal collaboration. Nor has she found a way for people to
advocate for themselves in meetings. But she recognizes the ethical
principle that people ought to participate in decision making about
themselves.

Rasha, too, describes how people are guided as collaborators in making decisions about actions that relate indirectly to goals. Brenda's goals (figures 3.2 and 3.3 in chapter 3) all appear to require management of daily living skills. However, these goals also require her to make decisions about when, how, and with whom she will act. Instead of managing people by doing the case coordination for them, Rasha describes how she works with people to coach them in making their own decisions about actions as simple as making phone calls:

Rasha Here, it's trying not to *do* [Rasha's emphasis] even phone calls for patients. When I worked in in-patients, we would often do the phoning for information on, say, a leisure club. Then, I'd give the patient the information. But here, we might do some preliminary calling to get an appropriate number of a person for the patient to talk to when they call. So, you're really trying to facilitate them doing every step ... so I might make a call to get some information – is this the number to call about such and such. OK, thank you. Then hand the number to the patient.

ET When would you consider that it would be useful to have them go through the steps of finding out that it was the wrong number?

Rasha We might observe their level of problem solving and their level of communication. For instance, Brenda might be an example of someone who's very concrete. But I think she can figure out who to call at what particular time – or where to look for a number – so I might let her do that – whereas John, for example, not only because of the language difficulty, but because of the whole communication style – I don't think the person on the other end would know what he was talking about – let alone if he had called the right place. I don't think he'd understand that or know what to do next. So, we're looking at problem solving, decision making and communication style.

Rasha contrasts her case coordination in mental health day programs with her previous work in 'in-patients.' Yet she continues to judge Brenda's ability to 'figure out who to call at what particular time – or where to look for a number.' With John, Rasha assumes that it is best not to leave him to find a telephone number because 'I don't think the person on the other end would know what he was talking about – let alone if he had called the right place.' Rasha later

explained that she encourages John to do what he can while supporting him so that he experiences success.

There is also evidence of collaborative decision making in planning the weekly program structure. Group planning meetings
encourage collaborative decision making around some aspects of the
program. They serve as a warm-up to greet people, check what is
happening, and tend to the interpersonal dynamics of the group.
Sometimes group sessions offer a collective forum for planning social
action. Another purpose of group sessions is to educate people in
decision making. People are asked to comment on the order of events
and the types of events on the program schedule. Where a group
decides to reorganize a schedule, participants, as often as professionals, reprint weekly sheets and change posted schedules. People are
also urged to suggest alternative locations for weekly outings, say, for
shopping, recreation, or visits to heritage or tourist sites. The organization of outings is negotiated to determine who will be involved,
where, who pays, and other arrangements. During decision-making
discussions, the professionals and some group members generally
ensure that everyone who wishes to has a chance to talk.

To account for the success of programs, those who attend are
encouraged to collaborate in program evaluation by commenting on
the program structure and their experience of specific programs.
Therefore, evaluation is not restricted to a professional perspective.
As people leave a program, they are often asked to comment on the
helpfulness of the program or their satisfaction in being treated 'as an
equal,' as shown in figure 4.1.

In all five areas, psychosocial rehabilitation programs pay particular attention to collaborative decision making, especially programs
that work from the Clubhouse or Fountain House models. Daily
check-in meetings are chaired by members. Members are encouraged
to express opinions and make choices on work projects, recreation,
and other aspects of the daily routine of programs; they are also
included in the development of program policies and may be co-
writers in requests for special grants funding. Professionals usually
speak publicly with members whose membership status appears to
encourage their participation in collaborative decision making with
professionals. The philosophy of psychosocial rehabilitation seems
to engender consciousness and action so that members and professionals actually challenge some provincial and federal practices that
limit collaborative decision making in structuring specific program

FIGURE 4.1
Client Satisfaction Survey (New Garden)*

Answer: always, sometimes, never

1 Case coordinator gave correct program information and descriptions.
2 The program components I am involved in are beneficial.
3 I can choose to change components when I feel I'm ready.
4 I feel that I am receiving the services offered to me at the time of admission.
5 My case coordinator treats me as an equal and shows concern and understanding toward me.
6 My case coordinator is there for me to discuss problems and concerns when I need to discuss them.
7 The staff teach me skills in order to reach my goals.
8 The staff teach me how to use resources in the community.
9 I have input into what my program will be.
10 My case coordinator and I discuss my progress in meeting my goals.
11 I use the skills I learn in my everyday life.
12 I am involved in planning my goals.
13 I learn new skills in the groups I attend.
14 Transportation to the program is a problem for me because of money, distance, fear.
15 Staff at the program help me feel comfortable in the program.
16 My case coordinator chooses my program goals.
17 The staff treat me as an equal and show concern and understanding toward me.
18 Clients have a say in how the program is run.
19 I have the opportunity to make my own choices/decisions.
20 I would recommend the program to someone in a situation similar to mine.
21 I know my program goals/rehabilitation.
22 I find it hard to follow the policies of the program (attendance, schedule, personal hygiene).
23 Staff are willing to talk with me about relationships.
24 I like the location of the program.
25 The program is a pleasantly furnished and well-maintained environment.
26 I can make a choice about a community placement when I am ready.
27 How helpful are the following types of treatment in your rehabilitation program? (fitness, individual counselling, personal effectiveness training, leisure/recreation, work units, peer support).

---

*Extracted from survey form

initiatives. Situations are analysed from the diverse perspectives of those attending programs, as well as from the perspectives of professionals; possible sequences of action and their implications are negotiated; and decision-making methods such as voting or taking turns in choosing are employed. People are asked to identify ideas, perspectives, and implications for various program options. Although occupational therapists and other professionals retain considerable control, the atmosphere is one of mutuality, respect for diverse perspectives and expertise, and some kind of involvement by everyone in decisions about day-to-day activities.

I was not surprised to see these examples since occupational therapists talk a lot about collaboration. Practice is often described as working *with* people rather than doing things *for* them. In fact, terms such as *collaboration* and *partnership* are common, as is reference to enabling people to develop *decision-making skills*. Canada's 1993 and 1997 guidelines, for occupational therapy's mental health and general practice respectively, emphasize collaboration throughout the full process of practice (Health Canada and Canadian Association of Occupational Therapists, 1993; Canadian Association of Occupational Therapists, 1997). Collaboration is linked to *client-centred practice*, and has been observed as a *mutual process of reasoning* or *collaborative reasoning* when professionals guide people in deciding goals and their implementation (Mattingly & Hayes Fleming, 1994).

Controlling Decisions Hierarchically

One can see and hear collaboration in everyday practice, until the breadth of decisions required to operate mental health services is considered. As chapters 2 to 7 show, reflection and analysis using the theory and method of institutional ethnography have brought into view the disjuncture of vision versus reality, of everyday experience versus ruling practices. If you trace collaboration in everyday practice to processes that organize power in decision making, you can see how hierarchy actually works.

Before proceeding, let us note that collaborative decision making is difficult to incorporate in mental health practice because some people have difficulties with decision making as part of their illness. When people experience psychoses, hallucinations, disturbing mood swings, or severe anxiety, decision making is clouded or actually impaired. As well, lack of experience in decision making, fear of making wrong decisions, assumptions of powerlessness, learned patterns of helplessness, and other personal barriers may make people reluctant to collaborate in making decisions. Even with the best of intentions, as Petra says,

we have to struggle with trying to get people to make as many decisions for themselves as we can without us having to take the leadership so that something actually does happen here.

Nevertheless, people with mental difficulties retain some decision-making capacity most of the time. Although professionals may doubt that people know what is best, people have their own view of what is best for themselves, based on their experience of living with mental health problems. Certainly, most people exhibit a strong desire to make choices and to exercise some degree of control in their lives. Besides, people learn subjectively how to work with professionals in mental health services, and they inherently know the organizational structure of mental health services because they have experienced it. This means that mental health problems are not sufficient justification for assuming that professionals are the only people who have expertise for making decisions about mental health services.

One can hear the tension of promoting collaboration within a medical hierarchy when occupational therapists talk about collaboration in the same breath as they talk or write about treating patients. By definition and classification, patients are not equal partners in deciding their diagnosis and treatment; instead, they are expected to rely on the expertise of a medical or psychological professional. Even if negotiation occurs, in the end, it is assumed that patients will accept professional judgment on the best treatment choices for a particular diagnosis or problem, so much so that it is common to hear people referred to as 'noncompliant' if they do not fit this assumed pattern. Moreover, professionals may face malpractice charges if people decide to take actions that contravene professional judgment, particularly if people harm themselves or others. Occupational therapists do share power in some decision making, but routinely organized barriers enable professionals and managers to control the basic structure of programs.

Many people have analysed barriers to collaborative decision making in mental health services; I wanted to know how decision making actually works. Dorothy Smith (1987) states that hierarchy is reproduced in *differentiations of policy- and decision-making capacities.* Her insight led me one afternoon to ask a group of eight people who were participants at Penrose what they would change about their day program. Without professional team members in the room (with the prior approval of professionals and the group), I asked what these peo-

FIGURE 4.2
Participants' Suggestions for Program Change (Penrose)

1 groups in the morning and activity in the afternoon with one-to-one time available in the afternoon
2 more explanation [from staff and people attending] so we know why we are doing things
3 staff and patients more a unit not two separate groups, e.g., lunch
4 more groups that actually teach you something
5 more organization of physical space

ple would change to make the program more ideal. As people talked, I prompted one person to write ideas on a flip chart using actual wording as much as possible. If an idea seemed like a duplicate, I asked the person expressing it to look at the list and decide if a point was already there. The point was added if there was any uncertainty that it had been covered. In about an hour, those present came up with five ideas that they wanted written on the chart (reproduced in figure 4.2). Then, a talkative group member called in the staff to listen to the ideas.

After listening, the staff members stated that they appreciated the ideas, found them useful, and would consider them at a professional staff meeting. At the meeting a few days later, the agenda included consideration of the five suggestions about the program. While staff members made reference to people's ideas, it was Petra who spoke up:

I understand that the group was saying that they don't feel that very much is happening here and I think we need to listen to that.

Despite Petra's attempt to legitimize people's ideas, she and the other professionals controlled decisions about the implementation of these ideas. In the end, the weekly schedule was adjusted. The psychologist started a new life skills group, including an action role-play session as a response to people's request for 'more groups that actually teach you something' (#4). Group times were shifted to the morning (#1). Time for 'activity in the afternoon with one-to-one time available in the afternoon' (#1) was scheduled. The professionals committed themselves to facilitate 'more explanation [from staff and people attending] so we know why we are doing things' (#2). One day a week was scheduled for professionals and program participants to eat lunch together (#3). And group members were invited to participate in the 'organization of physical space' (#5).

As I reflected on my invitation to people to list ideas for change, I became aware of decisions they had omitted. If directed to talk about a broader range of decision making, would these people have decided that psychiatric diagnosis and individual case management were appropriate mechanisms for enabling them to resolve their mental difficulties? Would they have decided that the quality and efficiency of professional practice should be based on their lives being managed as individual medical cases? Would they have decided that talking in group or individual sessions is more efficient than, say, working with an occupational therapist at home or at work?

The exercise is enlightening because we can actually see and hear the hierarchical relations between people who attend mental health programs and professionals: each professional and program participant reproduces the decision-making hierarchy of Canada's provincial mental health services. People's suggestions for changing the program structure fall within the decision-making boundaries marked out for them. They are welcome to suggest shifts in scheduling and in organizing space. Professionals are sympathetic with their displeasure at the separate eating habits of professional staff and program participants. Then professionals respond by deciding how to institute suggestions for changing some elements of the program structure.

Even when a vision of an ideal program is solicited, an invisible dividing line blocks participation in broader decision making. I feel confident that these people would have had ideas for making decisions about the broad program structure if asked specifically. But without prompting, their ideas did not trespass over an invisible boundary line. We are so used to existing structures that we do not question their presence or form. If we look more closely at the five areas that appear to be collaborative – program participation, personal goals, individual case coordination, personal preferences in the weekly program structure, and program evaluation – it becomes clear that the decision-making hierarchy of mental health services simultaneously invites yet confines collaboration.

First, I described people collaborating with professionals in making decisions about attending and participating in specific sessions within programs. Of course, some people prefer to rely on professional expertise, particularly if the professional is The Doctor. Petra knows that people still assume that professionals should control decision making and some people try to manipulate professionals by pretending that no one has informed them what to expect or do in programs:

We [professional team members] are increasingly realizing that the doctor just says [to people]: 'you're going to the program.' At first, we used to assume that people were just being manipulative in saying that they did not know what to expect. But I think it really is true that the doctor gives no real explanation, and they just arrive.

People choose whether or not to attend a program by deciding whether or not to comply with doctors' orders even if the 'doctor gives no real explanation.' Petra elaborates on the process of people's decision making about attending a program:

I suppose if you want to look at it in black and white, this is a voluntary program. So they've made the choice whether or not to come. If they've come, then we expect them to participate. And if they're not participating in the types of things we have, we find out why not. And if it's not something we want to change, we do suggest that they leave the program. Theoretically, once they choose to come to the program, people choose to be in all parts of the program. It's not, 'I'm going to take Parts A and B and leave the rest alone.' They are not deciding what group therapy is. They are, in that they are one of eight or nine people who have some impact on what the discussion is or what happens or whatever. But they don't decide that instead of group therapy, we're going to have an outing, or learning group, or whatever.

People are required to participate in decision making about access and admission to the program. Petra knows there are limitations on decision making because she points out that to choose to come to the program is to comply with the rules for participation. Staff 'expect' people to participate, and if they do not take part 'we find out why.' Staff will determine how to 'change' the program to suit those who decide to enter. But Petra is clear that the options for change are minimal: one takes or leaves the program as it is. Once in the program, people decide what 'impact' they will have on the group discussion, although they are 'not deciding what group therapy is' or whether 'we're going to have an outing, or learning group, or whatever.' In reality, people have so little control over program structure that they do not see themselves as leaders who might generate interest and enthusiasm about participation. I asked one group how people knew who would initiate discussion and what they would talk about. Wilma, who attends Penrose, replied:

This is the first time I've heard this – that we're supposed to get the ball rolling. I thought the staff were supposed to do that.

Collaborative decision making exists. Nevertheless, people's decisions are limited to choices about complying in programs. Wilma's response displays an awareness of the hierarchical order of decision making that excludes people from decisions about the program structure. Wilma displays the lived reality of choice in these programs: to comply or not with staff initiatives and the underlying structure.

And as Petra said above, people may decide their 'impact on what the discussion is or what happens.' But they do not decide what the sessions will be. The presence of a predetermined program structure controls decision making about the locations, time frames, philosophy, and funding that determine program sessions. When people were asked to comment on the program they were attending, their comments were about the organization of equipment and the division between individual and group time. The basic structure of a five-day, Monday to Friday, day program led by professionals in particular locations was not even raised for discussion.

Second, I described how people collaborate in setting their own goals for case management. Here again, we can see that collaboration is limited, in that the range of acceptable goals is implicitly controlled by the group design. Through observing peers, new cases implicitly learn that if they decide to name nonbehaviourial goals, or they identify goals for collective social action (figures 3.2 and 3.3), they may be out of line. As well, the locations, methods, and other features of groups are established by professionals who consider people's ideas as they did the suggestions generated during my session at Penrose. People are caught in a contradiction: they are expected to initiate group discussion, but only if it is relevant to individually diagnosed problems. On the one hand, professionals are educated in classes and practice settings to know what is relevant; on the other hand, people, like Wilma, are educated by experiencing the effect of services on their lives. Reflecting on Wilma's comment, Petra had a 'moment of ah ha' and asked, 'Are professionals actually interfering in what's supposed to happen in this group?'

Third, in regard to individual case coordination, Jill is an advocate for people making decisions about the management of their own cases. Unfortunately, people are not equal partners since they are categorized as cases, that is, as passive objects, rather than as active participants. People are not members of the case coordination team except by invitation from professionals. Professionals manage cases by deciding how much control people are capable of exercising in even basic activities such as making phone calls. As well, only professionals coordinate the management of all cases on a caseload. People may be individually included in case coordination meetings or medical rounds, but they attend simply to make comments on and hear decisions made about their own cases. Their decision making extends to their personal case, not to the management of caseloads and programs overall.

Fourth, I said that those who attend mental health day programs collaborate as participants in planning meetings. Yet planning, too, is carefully controlled. As described above, people are encouraged to be decision-making partners in deciding the day-to-day activities and topics of interest for discussion. However, they are only beginning to be included as decision-making partners on the committees, boards of directors, and other planning groups that control mental health services.

Fifth, since people are not members of the mental health team, they cannot be true decision-making partners in program evaluation. People contribute to consumer satisfaction ratings, but they do not define the questions or the rating scales. Furthermore, satisfaction ratings refer to the quality of people's everyday experiences in programs, without inviting evaluation of the quality of the program design, staffing, and funding allotted for programs. Although people's opinions have value in making specific programs accountable to those who attend, official decision making about the quality and efficiency of programs is based on the data collected through Management Information Systems (MIS). People are not partners in designing the MIS or in producing the MIS documentation. Nor are they involved in making funding decisions based on MIS documentation.

The barriers to collaborative decision making are considerable. At present, people do not even have observer or correspondent status on the team. Quite the contrary. Occupational therapy position descriptions, such as Rasha's (figure 3.1) require occupational therapists to take action, without reference to collaboration. It is the professional's duty to 'evaluate,' 'determine,' 'implement,' 'progress,' 'assess,' 'refer,' 'record,' and 'promote and practise good interpersonal and interdepartmental relationships.' Case coordinators (figure 3.4) are required to 'collaborate with the patient, team members, and significant others in order to establish priorities of care and to identify problems on an ongoing basis.' This statement confirms that collaboration is encouraged in determining priorities for individual action in case management. However, case coordinators, not those with mental health problems, are required to coordinate and control the multiple individuals who comprise a caseload.

In addition, professionals have privileges that are not available to the people who attend programs. The professionals at Penrose may choose whether or not to follow people's suggestions for program change (in figure 4.2). Professionals and managers can choose whether to be coffee break or meal partners with patients. Other privileges include having offices while those who attend programs do not; having shelves of texts and journals; being given paid time (and some refunds for expenses) to attend education sessions such as courses and workshops; and having access to institutional meetings and documentation that are out of bounds to patients. Professional privileges confine the extent of collaboration even when professionals intend to be collaborative.

It turns out that each example of collaboration has its boundaries. As Rasha says below, the team has responsibility to 'assign' and 'give histories.' The team is not currently open to full and equal partnership. Professionals 'assign' cases to each other and 'give' their histories to other team members who do not know them.

It's supposed to be really a case management meeting. In the sense that we will assign new cases and give histories if there have been new cases assessed or what have you.

Furthermore, Britte's comments clearly indicate that decision making about case coordination is controlled by the 'staff.'

This time is for the staff to meet to check in with each other – to touch base, to bring up questions, to make last-minute plans for the day, to organize to respond to what the day looks like, how many people appear to be showing up, who will and will not attend and what implications and demands that will have for the program.

Certainly people collaborate in managing their own cases. However when the team meets to coordinate work between cases, people need an invitation to join in. The invitation is for people to offer suggestions and advocate for their own ideas before professionals create the documentary (official) record. The official record turns collaborative discussions into professional decisions about the admission, participation, or discharge of cases. When I asked why people are not official team members, two dilemmas were usually raised.

One dilemma cited was that people's presence would decrease the decision-making efficiency required for case management. Mental health professionals perceive that the people who use their services would need to learn how assessment, admission, case management, team, and other policies and procedures work before they can make program decisions. Moreover, they argue, people diagnosed with mental disorders would need to learn how to document practice and cases in official records. Professional decision making is assumed to be quicker than collaboration because professionals know the method of case management. There is a view that it takes longer to collaborate, especially with those who are not professionally educated. Enabling people to become decision-making partners means educating them to develop and interpret institutional policies and decision-making practices. Underneath these arguments, it appears that mental health services value efficiency over equality in decision making.

The second dilemma raised about including people on the team was confidentiality. Professionals cite their codes of ethics and job requirements as guidelines for respecting the confidentiality of people being discussed. People are seen as having no comparable ethical guidelines. Realistically, professionals are still the only ones who are legally liable for breach of confidentiality, and thus for malpractice. Those who attend programs are not liable even if they are partners in group discussions or other forms of guidance. As yet, there is no official code of ethics for those categorized as patients.

Confidentiality restrictions present legal barriers that are not easily bridged. Legal requirements for controlling access to health records still prevent the use of this document as a vehicle for collab-

FIGURE 4.3
Policy on Confidentiality (Penrose)*

The primary purpose of the Health Record is to document the course of an individual's health care and to provide a medium of communication among those delivering health care. Unless both patient and practitioner can be assured that the Health Record will remain confidential, they may withhold information, thereby diminishing the value of the record and the quality of treatment.

Aside from the sharing of essential information by those people caring for the patient, there are three other ways in which information may be released:

1 Upon court order
2 Upon the written authorization of the patient
3 Upon request of a Minister of Health or agent

Any misuse of health information shall be considered a breach of confidentiality and shall be reported to the Executive Director. Disciplinary action will be taken up to and including termination of employment ... [followed by a section requiring staff to sign a Pledge of Confidentiality]

---

*Sample of the policy at Penrose

orative communication. A Policy on Confidentiality (figure 4.3) indicates that the 'primary purpose' of the health record is as 'a medium for communication.' However, it seems that the health record's more powerful 'primary purpose' is to protect professional and hospital liability should people bring professional charges or financial claims against the institution. Therefore, legal restrictions around confidentiality serve to control collaborative decision making since discussion of information is limited to 'those delivering health care.'

Professionals are legally prohibited from showing written information to anyone except for 'those people caring for the patient' on penalty of 'disciplinary action ... up to and including termination of employment.' Without signed consent, professionals cannot even reveal if someone attends a mental health program. Although confidentiality policies do not deliberately control collaboration, the threat of loss of a professional's employment serves that purpose. Professionals can summarize the essence of documents so that people know what has been written. However, the Right to Refuse Release of Information to patients (in Nova Scotia, but typical of other provinces) clarifies that:

the hospital or physician may refuse to make available patient medical

FIGURE 4.4
Program Description (Rosehill)*

[Rosehill Day Program] provides a short-term transitional program between inpatient [sic] and community living. In some cases it may provide a preventative service as an alternate to inpatient care for those requiring some support and intervention in community living skills. Home visits are an integral part of the program and the major focus is on health and community outreach.

Program planning is individualized providing:

1 behaviourial/functional assessments
2 skill development
3 involvement of significant persons in the patient's life
4 community integration
5 comprehensive discharge planning

*Sample from Service Manual

records if there are reasonable grounds to believe it would not be in the best interest of the patient. (extracted from the Right to Refuse Release of Information section of the Nova Scotia Hospitals Act, 1988)

It is the physician and other mental health professionals who sign approval for release of information; they, not 'the patient,' are officially designated to determine the 'best interest of the patient.' While confidentiality about people's personal situations must be respected, there is a need for some people with mental health problems to talk frankly about their experiences to educate ordinary people about mental health problems and diagnosable mental disorders. There is a dilemma here. We need people to speak publicly to educate us about their mental health problems, yet people who speak out about such difficulties may face discrimination if some landlords, employers, or others discover their mental health history, especially if people have seen psychiatrists.

Furthermore, the results of decision making about individual case management are reflected in hospital and provincial policies, procedures, and budgets, which are not seen by those who attend programs. Yet these are the documents used to make decisions about specific programs. An excerpt from a Service Manual in figure 4.4 describes a day program that was structured without any direct involvement from the people who attended the program. The decisions that this will be a transitional (day) program, involve medically diagnosed patients, and operate primarily through a system of individual case management may be appropriate but they have been made without participation from those who are supposed to benefit from these services.

Decisions about the locations, hours of operation, and salaries in mental health programs have to a large part been determined by the provincial government, hospital managers, union leaders, and professional representatives. Decision making about program philosophies is made by professionals and managers who decide the philosophic emphasis in each program. Decisions to support particular philosophic ideas and assumptions are not usually documented in the official minutes of government departments, but, rather, in professional texts and journals. The development of these philosophies is generally an academic and professional process that rarely includes those who use professional services.[2] Some provinces are changing mental health services. Mental health advisory boards within governments are including people as consumers, who then have access to decision-making discussions about policy development. This is an important development towards collaborative decision making. However, of the 24 members on the advisory board for one of the day programs in this study, none were consumers. As is typical of these boards, there are representatives from local mental health agencies, teachers' unions, barristers' societies, nursing associations, and other local hospitals. The only possibility for collaboration by those who use mental health services is by taking one of the three positions for member-at-large, little power to truly represent mental health consumers.

Now we can see that hierarchy is not merely an intellectual idea, but an everyday, ideological practice. In mental health services the hierarchy is sustained by categorizing people as patients in a dependent relation with professionals who control individual case management. Those who attend programs are allocated the power to make decisions about themselves and their immediate surroundings. Professionals, such as occupational therapists, occupy a middle layer of decision making about the philosophy, time, space, and other structural elements of specific programs. Occupational therapists collaborate in developing ideas about the day-to-day program structure and the team, and they are partners in making decisions about program schedules, types of group sessions, and people's access to services. Some occupational therapists, like Carol, sit on task forces or committees that are reorganizing provincial mental health services. However, decisions on such matters as assessment or case management have so far been out of bounds to most mental health occupational therapists. Upper levels of the hierarchy are controlled by provincial and federal government personnel, elected politicians, physicians, and lawyers who control the financial and legislative arrangements that guarantee the state's power to govern institutions.

In today's economy, the top hierarchical layer of control lies with international corporations, such as those that control medical insurance. Corporate insurance pays to treat individual pathology, not to enable the empowerment of those with mental health problems. Other corporate interests also support individualized, medically oriented mental health services, an outstanding example being the international pharmaceutical industry. Global competition in pharmaceutical and other industries means that countries like Canada are competing to produce goods as cheaply as places that provide low wages and few benefits to workers. International corporate control is now so great that national governments are being pressured to reduce the tax base for publicly funded programs, like mental health services.

Let us think now about commonly identified barriers and attempts to increase collaborative decision making in mental health services. The control of collaborative decision making is not merely an oversight that can be rectified by extending an invitation for people to join team meetings. As well, it is unacceptable to excuse mental health services from collaborative decision making on the justification that potential partners have mental health problems. While professional approaches may be experienced as barriers, we cannot move forward if we merely blame professionals for controlling mental health services through dominance, privilege, and arrogance. Certainly, we can point to barriers related to the patriarchal organization of mental health services, or inequities associated with race, class, age, sexual orientation, or other characteristic. But why does this organization persist?

To understand how hierarchy works and how it might be changed, we need to look at the routine organization of processes that account for quality and efficiency in individual case management. Efficiency is determined by the number of completed cases produced per month and year, not by the number of people who become decision-making partners in organizing mental health services. Two other routine forms of organization in mental health services stand out in controlling collaboration. One is decision making that requires prior knowledge of the policies and procedures of mental health services. The other is confidentiality policies that are linked to malpractice legislation. In reality, the ruling apparatus in mental health services is organized so that professional, managerial, and corporate interests intersect to determine how categorization, accountability, risk management, budgets, and legislation are hierarchically controlled. Control is exercised by the specific organization of mental health services, and by the provincial, federal, and international policies that determine what can be done in mental health services.

Hierarchical organization is diametrically opposite to the egalitarian, horizontal decision making required for empowerment. In differentiating decision-making capacities, hierarchy structures professionals to provide caregiving for dependent recipients. Those who invite individual and collective participation in decision making find themselves at odds not only with everyday situations, but with the overall organization of society. It is worth noting that hierarchical decision making and caregiving are not unique to health services. The modern world is organized hierarchically, from health services to religion to the military. Hierarchical relations are so embedded in society that historical examples of collaborating societies are forgotten, or discounted as heretical. If we are to move beyond today's dependence on professional and state caregiving, it is time to organize fully collaborating societies that both expect and guarantee citizen participation in all decision making.

5

Simulating Real Life

There is a popular expression that *knowledge is power*. It follows that empowerment (taking on power) is a process of learning. Empowerment education, facilitates a participatory process of learning to critique and transform individual feelings, thoughts, and actions, as well as the organization of society. This type of education involves learners as partners in both individual and collective action, the aim being to learn how power and resources can be shared equitably. Education generates knowledge about power, whether or not we are aware of being educated.

In recognizing that education can generate knowledge about power, I wanted to see what educational processes are included and omitted, funded and not funded in mental health day programs. I wondered how empowerment education is both practised and routinely organized, even though participants (learners) are transformed into psychiatric cases, collective action and social change are individualized in case management, and collaboration is controlled by hierarchical decision making. To this end, I decided to look at the curriculum that is displayed in the schedule of activities in day programs to see how people are learning, through simulations and real experiences, to live with or change life with a mental health problem.

Empowerment Education

A number of educators – Michael Apple, Brian Fay, Paulo Freire, Henri Giroux, Antonio Gramsci, Jack Mezirow, and Michael Welton, to name a few – have provided insights about the educational nature of enlightenment, emancipation, empowerment, and social justice. While they explore differing realms of life, they point to critical reflection, consciousness raising, conscientization (Freire), reflective reasoning, experiential learning, learning through doing, and real-life action as core educational processes in empowerment.

If empowerment is our goal, we need to organize education so that people learn how to reflect on and take action to change the organization of power in their lives. Since empowerment cannot be given to people, they need to learn from reflecting and doing, that is, to act reflexively. In other words, empowerment education must be person-centred (or learner-centred) in order to acknowledge that people have active power and the potential to reflect on and change the ways they live.

Empowerment education with adults has evolved mainly in Latin American and Asian countries, or in North American inner cities and aboriginal communities, where people are seeking ways out of poverty and oppression. The critical and transformative actions that characterize this type of education have emerged mostly outside formal school programs, and certainly outside mental health services. People with mental health problems have been involved in empowerment education in some circumstances, but almost never with health professionals, relying more on themselves or community activists. Without examples, I am on new ground in suggesting that mental health professionals could collaborate with those who have mental health problems to turn day programs into empowerment education.

Although there is no single design for an empowerment curriculum, one important part is critical reflection[1] on everyday life and on the organization of power. Empowerment depends on people becoming conscious of the invisible ways in which power is organized and embedded in everyday life. Critical reflection on power enables people, individually and collectively, to map a path for transforming their dependence into empowerment. The other part of empowerment education is experiential learning, which involves learners in real, bodily experiences. Experiential learning forms the basis for action and change towards empowerment. Critical reflection and experiential learning become intertwined as people acquire ideas, interests, attitudes, and skills that they deem relevant to their lives. Empowerment education facilitates learners to live, work, and play in all the occupations of real life. Individual reflection and skill development prepare people for collective action, such as participating in the organization of daily programming, and ultimately the organization of mental health services. Conversely, involvement in collective action builds both awareness and skills in individuals. The more that people diagnosed with mental disorders are educated to be active participants in organizing admission, case management, discharge, and other processes that intend to help them, the more they will think of themselves as empowered and develop the competence to be empowered people. By integrating critical reflection and real experiential learning, people will learn through what Kolb (1984) and others have described as reflection-in-action.

To facilitate reflection-in-action is to facilitate consciousness-raising and participatory processes of learning. Lectures and other class-based lessons are used if people indicate (on their own or by suggestion) that they want to hear specific information or a particular perspective. Lecturing and laboratory exercises can be used to engage participants in listening or simulation-based learning. These methods are useful to alert people to ideas, or new skills. However, they intellectualize learning – learning that needs to extend into reflection and action in real life. Therefore, empowerment educators, who may be professionals or not, facilitate, guide, coach, encourage, support, prompt, stimulate, acknowledge, and otherwise engage people as reflective, active participants.

Beyond the day-to-day curriculum, structures and organizations need to support empowerment education. For instance, possibilities for education are influenced by the ways in which space and time are organized. Empowerment education may begin in simulated places and fixed schedules that create a protective learning environment away from the distractions and complexities of real life. When this type of learning is needed, simulation exercises can involve people in the *codification* of their experiences in designated educational settings. Codification (a term borrowed from Freire) simulates real situations in dance, pictures, role-play, drama, music, or other creative forms. The situation is *coded* – that is, interpreted – so that power is brought into view for analysis. For instance, the group of people who identified five changes they would like to see in Penrose day program could act out a scene in which professionals eat at a large, central table while people who attend programs eat at small tables on the periphery. Such a scene could be role-played in a classroom to prompt discussion about the marginalization people experience and about possible actions for their integration in real situations. Codification helps people to visually and physically unravel the personal and organizational features that shape their lives (Freire, 1985).

Codified learning through simulations needs to be transferred into real-life places and times. In other words, empowerment education must be structured so that learning extends into the real situations that people face; empowerment cannot be learned solely in a classroom setting or in artificial time schedules. This kind of education seizes real opportunities to prompt critical reflection on power and action. Locations and schedules for empowerment education need to be flexible rather than standardized in order to offer a range of simulation and real experience, as well as life-long individual and collective learning about the self and society.

Guiding Critical Reflection and Experiential Learning

If one casually observes mental health day programs, the curriculum actually looks as if it includes reflection and action, the two important parts of empowerment education. Moreover, facilitation, coaching, encouragement, demonstration, discussion, and other enabling methods are used far more than lectures or classroom sessions. In fact, adult mental health day programs are not usually recognized as legitimate sites for adult education: they occur outside of designated places of education, and only sometimes use a classroom model of education.

To get beyond casual observation, we need to examine the program curriculum and methods in the locations (space) and schedules (time) in which they occur. One can *see* the organization of space by noting the actual locations, facilities, and equipment of everyday practice. We already know that people are expected to participate in the weekly schedule offered through mental health day programs. Schedules appear to encourage individual and collective action, even though programs are accountable primarily for individual case management. Facilities, too, are designed for both individual and group sessions. Time is included for people to collaborate in structuring specific program activities even though they are excluded from decision making about the overall structure of mental health services. We still need to ask whether program locations are designed for simulating or engaging in real life and whether schedules include time for critical reflection and experiential learning relevant to people's real lives.

The programs in hospital settings are located away from in-patient wards. They occupy a floor, a wing, or a set of rooms that distinguish the space as a separate unit. Access to the four hospital-based programs in this study is not direct from outdoors. People have to go through various hospital sections to reach the day program area. Some programs are located in houses in or near residential areas. The two house-based programs in this study have facilities and equipment that more or less resemble the homes, recreation areas, and workplaces of at least some people's real lives. All programs have some office space and group rooms with flip charts and tables for professionals and people to critically reflect on their experiences and on the organization of power. To a varying degree, program space is designed with kitchens, lounges, workshops, washrooms, handcraft areas, recreation rooms, clerical work areas, maintenance storage areas, and halls where people can learn through experience. Programs are all accessible by public transportation.

Weekly schedules, posted near the entrances to the program space, generally describe the Monday to Friday array of activities, which I have labelled as 'interactional' and 'occupational' sessions in figure 5.1. I have used the term 'interactional sessions' to describe sessions that emphasize discussion or verbal counselling, and 'occupational sessions' for those that are experiential, involving people in a wide array of occupations, viewed broadly as everything people do to occupy life.

Programs are typically scheduled to start at 9:00 a.m. and finish at 3:00 p.m. Occupational therapists generally work from 8:00 or 8:30 a.m. to 4:30 or 5:00 p.m. They gain considerable flexibility by including some evenings and weekends to respond to changing program events and people's specific needs. Mental health professionals generally fill daytime positions covered by hospital (or government) and union agreements. Overtime is informally organized without salary adjustments. There are breaks mid-morning and mid-afternoon, with an hour usually designated for lunch.

As well, depending on the organization of space, there is time for real experiences in such occupations as meal preparation, recreation, handcrafts, outings, 'doing for others,' and community involvement. People who attend mental health day programs become involved in

FIGURE 5.1
Core Curriculum: Interactional and Occupational Sessions*

	Interactional	Occupational
Bayview	Personal growth Life skills Group therapy Stress management Communication group Assertiveness training Individual sessions	Group meal Activity (handcrafts) Lunch preparation Recreation Individual sessions
Clearcove	Verbal group Stress management Individual sessions	Activity (handcrafts) Bowling Individual sessions
Jackson Heights (psychosocial rehabilitation)	Individual sessions	Life skills Work skills Work therapy Outreach work therapy Hospital industries Handcrafts Recreation Outings
New Garden (psychosocial rehabilitation)	Personal effectiveness training (P.E.T.)	Food services Clerical Maintenance Recreation Outings
Penrose	Group therapy Creative expression Life skills Values Stress management Individual sessions	Cooking Activity (handcrafts) Lunch preparation Games (Friday group only) Music Outings Individual sessions
Rosehill	Health & lifestyle Stress management Assertiveness training Individual sessions	Aerobics Doing for others Aquacize Individual sessions Community day

*Table constructed from weekly schedules and observation notes. There is no program schedule at Merrivale.

decorating and cooking for Christmas and preparing special meals for other events. Some planning time is used for preparing menus, shopping, and other aspects of these events.

New Garden typifies the usual organization of space and time in a mental health clubhouse. More than in psychoeducation programs, the vast majority of time is spent in the real occupations needed to operate these programs: food services, clerical work, and maintenance. People shop in real stores and cook, set tables, wait on tables, clean up, and check supplies associated with real coffee breaks, lunch, and supper. Those doing clerical work do the photocopying, collating, typing, and other clerical duties required by these programs. Maintenance work includes painting, lawn-mowing, snow-shovelling, repairs, and other duties that keep up program facilities. Other occupations in a mental health clubhouse are gardening, recycling, or mail duties, which contribute to the running of the clubhouse. Time is organized to provide an educational program based on the real routines and tasks that sustain and develop a clubhouse. As I have already indicated, members of clubhouses are involved in real public processes such as voting and speaking publicly about mental illness or about transportation, job training, and other issues that affect them as citizens.

Every mental health day program includes time for 'outings' in real community settings (e.g., swimming, badminton, bowling). There are also outings to malls or other places of interest, such as a museum or radio station. Real situations are viewed, in part, as an assessment opportunity, as Petra describes:

I think of the times, say we've been on an outing, and we're coming back, and I'll say to somebody, 'Boy, did you see how so-and-so participated, or did you see what so-and-so did or said to me?' or whatever I think is a reflection of whatever difficulty they've come in with. Whereas, at other times when I've done a group on self-esteem or assertiveness or whatever, we often find we're not coming out of that group any more enlightened about people. Or without having offered them any more than when they went into it.

Petra indicates that seeing people in real situations makes her 'more enlightened about people.'

Some real situations are seized as opportunities to facilitate learning relevant to the moment, as Jill describes (the lesson is on using a phone book):

I see myself as a teacher. But not in the formal sense. By taking advantage of an opportunity as it arises, it can be a very spontaneous thing. Sometimes you might have a set schedule to teach somebody something. But if someone comes up with a problem, for example, and they need to contact somebody, I would naturally capitalize on that and say, 'Here's the phone book.' And they might say 'You call.' And right away, I'll say, 'No, I won't. OK, can you look up a number in the phone book? Here's how you do it.' So, I think in every-day situations we capitalize on those opportunities. And they are often the best ones. They are the ones that are important to that client at the time. If I sat down with that client the next day and said 'Here's how to use the phone book,' he'd say 'Right, I've got better things to do.'

Occasionally, occupational therapists go to people's homes and community situations to educate them in the instrumental skills of community living. As Jill says:

If we need to tutor their ability to function in the house – learning how to use the washer and dryer or something like that – something more lifeskills or community living skills related – for example, using the bus – we would actually go out and do that.

This is in marked contrast with health practices, where professional time is organized into a linear series of appointments for care, special tests, consultation, or counselling. Time in mental health day programs is structured from an educational perspective to mirror the multiple demands of real nine-to-five jobs. Individuals and groups are engaged in experiential learning to some degree. Learning occurs in real occupations, including those through which people look after themselves, enjoy life, and make some social if not economic contribution to society. People complete real projects related to special events. Or they do the real work of feeding people and looking after the clerical and maintenance work that has a real, meaningful function in operating a program.

Having asked initially how much day programs resemble empowerment education, I found that they incorporate reflection and action in important ways that make them quite different from typical health services. One day Rasha told me that mental health day programs feel like true occupational therapy, as it is supposed to be practised, even though there is often only one occupational therapist in each day program.[2]

Educating through Standardized Simulations

Knowing that power is invisibly embedded in everyday situations, I needed to go beyond observation to understand the possibilities for empowerment education. Since I was exploring points of tension, I wondered if there is a line of fault in which day program education generates knowledge for empowerment while the routine organization undermines empowerment. Dorothy Smith's view of a bifurcated consciousness is that contradictory processes can occur simultaneously without awareness because the organization of these processes is 'extra-local,' invisible, and beyond consciousness yet embedded in routine, taken-for-granted ways of conducting everyday life.

When I began to trace program activities to organizational features, the analysis revealed a central element of the tension experienced by occupational therapists: occupational therapy discourse and practice display this profession's intentions and actual successes in educating people with mental health problems to live as fully as possible; but occupational therapists who work in mental health day programs separate people from real life and rely on people's learning through a limited range of simulated experiences that may not resemble their real life. You heard at the beginning of the book how Petra experiences this tension:

I've had this activity background – this occupational therapy background; but so many of the things that I've found myself doing here, I'm not trained for.

Petra recognizes that involving people in 'activity' is not what is really required of her, while Britte experiences this as being 'not very clear on the role ourselves.' Although occupational therapy is derived from the occupational work done in nineteenth-century asylums in England and France, practice has been greatly restricted in modern hospitals, which are subject to labour laws; patients are protected from exploitation, and union jobs cannot be done for free. Hospitals have had to confine education programs to simulated experience so as to avoid competing with union labour.

It is important here to remind ourselves that people attend mental health day programs because they are having difficulty living real life. Given that real life presents some complex and hard-to-solve problems, there is value in at least temporarily simulating real life in a protected, safe environment with sympathetic group members and professionals. In fact, mental health day programs are often classified as *transitional*; their purpose is to offer learning that is, as Carol says,

a sort of transition point between being in hospital and being functional again in the community.

Programs function as a bridge that Carol describes as touching both hospital and community life. If the purpose of these programs is transitional education, then one would expect professionals to guide people through transitions during simulation as well as real experiential learning. However, the transitional purpose is not the only driving force behind mental health day programs. Some policy documents describe these as *partial-hospitalization* programs, a title suggesting that day programs may be a bridge, but they are also a form of management that reduces the cost of hospital services. Occupational therapy job and program descriptions do not restrict occupational therapists from practising in real community situations. However, during my 74 days of observation, I saw only four visits to personal residences or group homes: two by Petra and two by Rasha, whom I observed for eight and six weeks respectively. As Neva says:

One of the things that might interfere ... with the notion of empowerment ... is the connection with the hospital. I think that's something. Because that keeps you quite attached to the medical model although you're trying to work with something that's very different.

While practice occurs in real kitchens, workshops, and so forth, the location, facilities, and equipment are all simulations of people's real-life circumstances. As well, simulations represent only a small segment of real life. Selected simulations may be relevant to some but not all of the people who attend these programs. As Neva says, the structure is determined by the program connection with hospitals that operate from a 'medical model.' She highlights: 'you're trying to work with something that's very different.'

Critical reflection and experiential learning are most constrained in the mental health day programs that are organized in urban hospitals. Rather than practise simulation activities, those from rural areas may need to learn to address difficulties in organizing or finding meaningful, paid part-time work if they live far from public transportation and those from urban areas may need to learn to ask for help or build a social network so that they can live in a boarding-home and use local buses. Clerical, woodworking, cooking, and maintenance equipment in clubhouse programs are not necessarily similar to the real work situations that some people face outside programs. The group discussion rooms and mini-kitchens in hospital-based programs may be entirely irrelevant to people's real lives.

The locations and equipment of mental health day programs seem suitable for reflection and simulated, experiential learning. Although one can attend to people's real lives, one can do so primarily by simulating only one version of reality. As Britte says:

[a woman attending a program] needs to practise being in a social situation – going out in the community and actually looking for work. I can practise it in here till the cows come home. But I can't go out there right now. Or maybe we need another occupational therapist whose job is community work.

The 9:00 a.m. to 3:00 p.m. period represents a real work schedule for some people, but certainly not all. For example, a regular, daytime, five-day structure is not real to homemakers, parents, shift workers, or self-employed persons. These people determine their own hours or respond to people's needs at various hours. As well, the time schedule resembles a work day. But many people raise problems related to personal care, leisure, and general community occupations that occur at various times of the day or night and are unrelated to work. In essence, time, like space, is structured to represent only a small segment of real life that is relevant to only some people.

Program Philosophies

At this point, I found myself asking why space and time in mental health day programs are structured to simulate singular versions of real life. To answer this question, I traced space and time to two less visible organizational processes, namely the selection of a *program philosophy* and *funding*.

First let us look at the two main philosophies underlying mental health day programs in Atlantic Canada: psychoeducation and psychosocial rehabilitation.

Psychoeducation

Five programs were based on psychoeducation and included varying amounts and types of interactional and occupational sessions: Bayview, Clearcove, Merrivale, Penrose, and Rosehill day programs.

The philosophy of psychoeducation structures programs around ideas and beliefs that psychological education can enable people to better attend to their own mental problems. Briefly summarized, this is an educational approach that involves people in learning to cope with and adapt to life with mental health problems. Psychoeducation is based on a biopsychosocial model of mental health. As the name implies, psychoeducation focuses on educating people about psychological processes and their influence on behaviour. It promotes an information-based, intellectual form of learning through simulation of the real behaviour associated with interpersonal and group interaction, and with personal growth. As Rasha says,

[we] tend to think of information as empowering. So the more information on assertiveness or stress management a person has, the better.

While including some occupational sessions, psychoeducation programs emphasize interactional sessions, notably personal growth, life skills, assertiveness training, stress management, and communications, as listed in figure 5.1. Interactional sessions offer individual and group counselling in which simulation exercises are often used as a stimulus for thinking about and reflecting on real life. There is an interplay between reflection and simulated experience, although the translation of learning from simulated to real-life experience and situations is left largely to the person.

Carol describes how she engages people in 'activity' as a 'measuring stick' of psychological progress.

I always explain the use of activity as a kind of measuring stick that they can utilize to determine if their medications are helping – if their concentration is improving or if they are beginning to even feel like coming to activity. I explain that, at first, you don't even feel like you want to come. Then you'll be able to come for ten minutes. Then you'll notice that you can do fifteen minutes, then a half-hour. I try to give them control and help them to see how they can use it. And then that's followed up by our activity laboratory questionnaire that I showed you – where they score themselves on how they are improving in activity. And then, from there, get them involved. I've managed to refer some people to other activities just to get some involvement in the community.

She does not indicate whether she facilitates critical reflection or the transfer of experiential learning in 'activity' into real life. What Carol does say is that activity is part of assessment, part of her management of individual cases. Besides its use in assessment, activity is used as a medium for developing psychological traits such as 'concentration.' She is engaging the person in experiential learning. But she appears to be using 'activity' as a tool for the assessment and therapeutic components of case management in a hospital context where opportunities to involve people in real life are not available.

In another situation, Rasha facilitates Brenda's reflection on her real life in which she needs to 'take medication.' Paper and pencil exercises are commonly used to create lists, charts, diagrams, and other visual representations of imaginary or remembered situations. Or people may represent their living space by drawing their homes or community situations. Drawing may also be used to symbolize relationships, emotions, or thoughts. To get information on Brenda's use of medication, Rasha asks her to simulate her weekly activities by representing what she does, including taking medication, on a schedule. Brenda represents her real life on paper by filling in a sheet drawn with seven columns, three sections to a column, representing morning, afternoon, and evening segments of the week.

Simulations provide bodily experience and create tangible objects for reflecting on real life without real involvement. In themselves, these approaches are creative, insightful ways of prompting critical reflection through codification, the method advocated by Paulo Freire for empowerment education. The use of simulated action enables people to visualize and talk about their real lives in a safe situation. People may also develop skills that potentially can be transferred to real-life situations. Missing in these psychoeducation programs, however, are sufficient opportunities for people to transfer their codified learning into real-life experience. For instance, psychoeducation programs typically include assertiveness sessions that follow a fairly standardized process, like the following:

1 staff or groups members reviewing concepts of assertiveness
2 group members in turn discussing a specific situation during the past

week when they felt angry, helpless, frustrated, impatient, overlooked, overwhelmed, bored, scared, punished, criticized unfairly, and so on.

3 some group members engaging in a role-play to recreate a situation
4 discussing assertiveness issues as group members see them, with ideas contributed by staff
5 re-creating the role-play following guidelines for being assertive
6 defining a behaviourial objective for practising assertiveness over the next week (sometimes called 'homework')

One variation is to have a group work with a particular theme or emotion. The theme might be frustration, where each group member defines a real situation in which frustration has been or continues to be experienced. A few people volunteer to role-play remembered then revised versions of real frustrating situations. They do so in the simulated conditions of programs and with group members who are not the real people involved in the frustrating situation. Those who are observing the role-play may engage in discussion and reflection on their own situation or that of someone else. At the end of the day everyone physically leaves the program to return to their real lives. With them are memories of observing a role-played experience and of talking about frustration.

While psychoeducation programs emphasize the dialogic forms of codification that are consistent with empowerment education, learning is largely through representation in situations that are removed from real life. The situations are remembered rather than real. I observed Andrea, a person in the assertiveness group at the Rosehill day program, commenting on the importance she places on the program's linking of reflection to real life:

I had been through assertiveness and stress management groups on the in-patient unit. But I must say I found that I've learned things in the groups here. You do them differently. And you run and approach these groups differently. I found that I learned quite a few things. I really learned things that were practical for my life.

The point here is that role-plays may positively address people's real-life situations, but they are based on interpretations rather than shared, real experience. No other group members were present in the real situations, so that they cannot respond with knowledge of those situations. They can only respond to people's interpretations of real situations in a different context. Conversely, group members transfer learning from the group to real situations. However, what enters and leaves these sessions is a remembered, interpreted version of real life and a memory of role-plays. These multiple realities are not brought together in the same space and time. Furthermore, the main interpreter is a person who has been diagnosed with a mental disorder because of difficulties in managing, perceiving, or interpreting everyday life. As far as the possibilities for professionals to involve people in empowerment education are concerned, professionals and other group members are absent in the actual transition between real and simulated space and time. They can neither corroborate nor refute interpretations that people have made as they attempt to translate their learning from simulated situations in the program to real life.

We can appreciate that Brenda's weekly goals (in figure 3.2) are real to her: do laundry, do dishes nightly, cut friend's hair. However, Rasha prompts Brenda to translate these everyday life goals into assertiveness goals using the standardized format for setting assertiveness goals in psychoeducation programs. Therefore, Brenda defines her assertiveness goals as 'making positive statements' and 'giving compliments,' as listed in figure 3.3. Brenda is asked by Rasha to reflect in the group on the 'homework' she chose in the previous week to address assertiveness goals. She reflects on a goal defined as 'making requests,' a standard goal for many people in this program:

Rasha   Have you been making requests?
[Note: Brenda's 'homework' was to 'make one request per day' as articulated by the therapist from Brenda's discussion the previous week about her difficulty speaking up and asking for help when she felt overwhelmed, and the feelings grew into helplessness, panic, mania, and fear of hospitalization.]

Brenda   I don't know. I guess I made a request to my son. I asked him to clean up the living room. And I was just amazed he did it in no time. I gave him a compliment and said thank you. [As Brenda talked, her face became more and more animated. She smiled and leaned forward in her chair. She had more expression. Her voice was stronger.] He comes in the door and just throws everything down, his school bag and everything. You come directly into our apartment into the living room and he treats that like his own room. I guess that's like any teenager. I said to him 'I'm just looking around this room. Are you looking around too? Are you going to clean it up?' He said OK and had it done in a few minutes.

Rasha　It sounds like you did your homework after all. Now what would you like to try this week?

Rasha does not attempt to facilitate real experiential learning. Rather, she teaches Brenda to reflect on her real life in a location separate from real life. She also teaches her to think about her life using the behaviourial definitions of assertiveness used in psychoeducation. The aim is for Brenda to develop skills to reflect on her behaviour in real life and to engage in new psychologically defined behaviour within simulated conditions.

Rasha did visit Brenda's home on one occasion. Apart from this, the transitional learning was left for Brenda to do on her own without Rasha's guidance. As she role-plays making compliments in a group session, Brenda makes real compliments to real people sitting in the group. But these are not the people Brenda faces in her real life. The role-plays are an intellectual interpretation made by Brenda and those who hear her story. They are abstract, reasoned versions of what really happened and might happen in Brenda's real life. As Brenda participates in recreation, she is encouraged to make compliments and requests so that the idea is integrated with real action. Once again, the swimming and aerobics that Brenda does for recreation are real, but they are not what she does in real life. These activities may teach her to enjoy such recreation and plan to include it in her real life, but she is still left to translate that experience and organize it without the same intensity and sophistication of guidance provided by health professionals for the intellectual part of her learning.

This analysis displays another piece of the ideological circle of case management. The emphasis on simulation is organized in the routine approaches used for the psychological education of mental cases. Case management is based on the creation of mental facts that are first interpreted as diagnostic categories, then shaped into another set of facts called goals. Goals interpret lived reality in terms of mental constructs such as assertiveness, stress, and so on. We can see that simulation exercises, such as role-plays and paper and pencil exercises, attempt to change people's reality using mental goals as an interpretative framework. The framework authorized to justify and

organize this practice is the philosophy and practice of psychoeducation. This type of educational practice simulates life experience as a
method of educating individually diagnosed cases to demonstrate
change in behaviourial goals. The circle is completed by using textual facts about progress on goals to demonstrate the quality and efficiency of practice in psychoeducation programs. Psychoeducation is
efficient since it provides a way for mental health professionals to
work with more people in groups than could be done individually. In
spite of their patient classification, people learn to participate in
their own healing and re-education, at least as individuals and as people who can live with this kind of support in their own communities.
It seems that psychoeducation is a means of reducing hospital costs
without educating people so extensively that they learn to collectively challenge the hierarchical organization of professional forms
of mental health practice and organization.

Psychosocial Rehabilitation
In contrast with psychoeducation, the philosophy of psychosocial
rehabilitation (PSR) structures programs around ideas and beliefs
that mental disorders result from social as well as biological and psychological factors. There is strong recognition that mental health
problems influence and are influenced by real-life experience.[3] The
emphasis is on educating people to develop the instrumental skills
needed for everyday living. Psychosocial rehabilitation is an
umbrella term under which people talk about the Fountain House
model, or the Clubhouse model. Psychosocial rehabilitation advocates that people are 'members' who control their own goal setting in
a system of individualized case management, with attention to social
circumstances, as well as individual behaviour. The philosophy takes
into account that people are struggling with real-life difficulties such
as poverty, a poor employment history, limited skills for living, a
small network of social support, and the social stigma that local
neighbourhoods attach to them. In this study, Jackson Heights and
the New Garden day programs follow a psychosocial rehabilitation
philosophy most closely, although all programs adhere to this
approach to some extent. The New Garden day program is strongly
based in psychosocial rehabilitation, relying almost solely on occupational sessions. The Jackson Heights day program emphasizes psychosocial rehabilitation and occupational sessions, but is not fully
developed as a mental health clubhouse.

My summary of psychosocial rehabilitation is highly simplified. In actual practice, there are many versions. Some psychosocial rehabilitation programs are behaviourial, with organized schemata for the incremental development of skills. Many clubhouses exclude professionals altogether and operate on private funding. Others operate through professional–member partnerships, particularly if funding is from the public purse. New Garden Clubhouse is publicly funded and administered through a hospital mental health service. A professional–member partnership has organized work units within facilities as well as units for employment, housing, and other elements of real life.

The schedule in psychosocial rehabilitation features occupational sessions (as in figure 5.1) that emphasize experiential over intellectual learning. The program content is weighted away from simulation exercises and discussion, and toward real cooking, house cleaning and maintenance, telephone reception and message taking, basic clerical duties, and basic employment skills in industrial subcontracted work projects such as recycling and packaging. These occupations are real in that people are handling materials that they fashion into products for real purposes.

Although facilities and schedules appear more real than in psychoeducation programs, the occupational sessions in psychosocial rehabilitation are still organized in facilities and with equipment that simulate a singular version of real life. For instance, I observed Neva working with Hal around meal planning, shopping, kitchen organization, and cooking:

9:22 a.m.:
Neva asks Hal, who is chef for the day, to sit down in the dining area to go over the menu for the noon meal before they go shopping and before Hal talks to the other people he will be directing that day in the kitchen.

Neva I've changed your menu here ... I've substituted mashed potatoes for the rice, and cottage cheese for the hard cheese in the salad in order to cut costs because our costs are getting up there ... Sometimes with a menu like this we have to compromise one thing for another, so since you have pork chops, I took off the cheese and rice ... this is a very good menu ... What you need to do now is fill out the tasks cause you'll be running the meeting to help the rest of the group get organized in a few minutes ... so what tasks need to be done? [Hal took the sheet and pen and started to make a list]. You're right [when Hal wrote down 'make bran muffins'] ... then what else? [Hal said 'make pork chops'] ... Yes, that's right, but you can break it down so that you put here that someone browns the pork chops and puts on sauce because then we'll do them in the oven.

Hal and others are preparing for a real meal. Neva facilitates action by helping Hal to plan to take on real supervisory duties. The action itself is real rather than role-played. Neva is very directive; nevertheless, reflection is elicited during conversations in which she asks Hal questions such as 'So what did you think of that?' and 'What do you need to know to live on your own?' and 'Where will you get money to support yourself?' Questions elicit reflection on everyday life in which real action is taking place.

Situations like the one described with Hal show how some programs educate people to live in artificially organized space and time. The action does not occur in Hal's real apartment, rather it occurs in a simulated kitchen. While the cooking and kitchen are real, Hal's boarding-house kitchen has far less equipment and fewer supplies. He will also be managing on a far stricter food budget than is available even in financially strapped mental health programs. People are learning to make nutritious food. We know that the pork chops and muffins may still be beyond the budget or cooking conditions that people like Hal face at home. Neva can go to Hal's apartment occasionally, but her caseload and work responsibilities make home visits generally impractical.

Psychosocial rehabilitation programs look like empowerment education. They generally educate people through real experience far more than do psychoeducation programs. Let us not forget, though, that meal planning and other occupations inside program facilities are simulated versions of real experience. Hal, like Brenda, is translating reflections from his home experience into action in a simulated facility.

It appears that the philosophies of psychoeducation and psychosocial rehabilitation both organize day programs to promote basic life skills, whether they be in relating to others or cooking, in protected, simulated one-on-one or group situations. The design and schedule have potential for educating people in collective action to transform their marginalized lives, but we have already seen that assessment and admission, individual case management, and controlled decision-making processes interact to narrow education to individual concerns with instrumental living. Psychosocial rehabilitation programs are most likely to prompt some learning about collective action, but their perspective is focused on actions for sustaining a positive, self-contained refuge in the midst of a stigmatizing, marginalizing society.

Funding

Now I asked why programs rely on philosophies that educate people mainly through simulation. I decided to trace the educational curriculum to processes of funding. It seems that budget categories, petty cash, and revenue-generation processes leave professionals little choice but to emphasize simulation over real action. The emphasis occurs regardless of whether the philosophy is psychoeducation or psychosocial rehabilitation, although psychoeducation programs are increasingly supporting people in regular housing, employment, and recreation.

Approximately 97 per cent of mental health day program funding is for salaries. Typically, salaries pay for a single team that operates during daytime hours. It is unusual to have funding for other teams that might work early in the day, late in the evening, or in real community situations, although the New Garden day program is moving rapidly in this direction. Practices that are grounded in real situations usually must be covered by staggering the work schedules of existing team members. Some relief is offered by providing time off in lieu of overtime work. Otherwise, staff volunteer extra time to make the program work. Not only do salaries structure staff time, but they structure program possibilities. There are almost no funds for the actual program. Day programs generally include a budget category called 'occupational therapy supplies' or 'activity supplies.' Some include a category for 'outings' or 'recreation.' However, the amounts are all taken out of the 3 per cent or so allocated for nonsalary items. Together, occupational therapy supplies, recreation, and outings are allocated no more than a few thousand dollars per year. We should acknowledge that the presence or absence of occupational therapy supplies in a budget can be misleading. New Garden, for instance, does not include occupational therapy as a budget item. Rather, materials for the food services, clerical, and maintenance units are funded (minimally) as necessary items for the day-to-day running of the program.

Another funding mechanism is petty cash, which tends to operate as a separate budget envelope from that for salaries and supplies. In all programs, petty cash is used to purchase real-activity supplies or to buy materials for small revenue-generating projects. This is particularly true in Jackson Heights and New Garden day programs. Food, crafts, and other products not only sustain the program but are made for sale (see the description of revenue generation below). Hospital-based programs are inclined to use the hospital purchasing system where policies, like at Rosehill, indicate that staff are not to resort to petty cash unless this is 'therapeutically appropriate,' as if this would be an unusual situation:

Food required for patient treatment programs may be requisitioned from the Food Services Department.

If therapeutically appropriate or if foodstuffs unavailable from Food Services, items may be purchased outside.

Staff requiring bus tickets for business or patient programs must obtain authorization.

The general policy is to use the specialized buying and transportation systems organized by hospitals. These policies may increase efficiencies in using bulk orders that reduce the cost of supplies. But this routine practice is to reduce the potential for people to learn to budget real money and buy food in real stores. Despite the presence of policies for limiting outside buying, each program allocates from $50 to $200 per expenditure of petty cash to cover small-outing costs, and to purchase handcraft materials or food for cooking. In this way, petty cash provides flexibility and spontaneity for real community experiences. But the funding for this type of work is minuscule. Given this limited financial support, possibilities for real action are small-scale.

As Petra says, petty cash allows people to do a few ordinary things in the community like going out for a meal or bowling:

Three to four dollars per person for a meal out – equal to meal tickets in the cafeteria. I ask for $30 for groceries and $20 for an outing unless I know it will be more or less expensive ... [re outings] When we started, we tended to do a lot of bowling, which is more costly, but we've been doing trips which are cost-free like the radio station ... We've had suggestions that we go horse-back riding. But at $10–12 per person, what we do is say to people that's beyond our budget, let's try to do a fundraiser if you want to do something special like that ... I don't have any written guidelines but anything that's in excess of $5 per person, we'd have to think about or do some more fundraising.

As my observation notes of the Bayview day program indicate, the standard budget includes very few materials, so that petty cash and just plain scrounging are used to provide opportunities for engaging people in real handcrafts:

Projects are chosen by the occupational therapist and occupational therapy assistant if they require very little material, can be completed within vary-ing levels of skills, and are designed for short-term completion. The assis-tant chooses things from craft catalogues and orders the materials so that inventory, to a large degree, determines what activities are available to do ... they use local, donated materials where possible. The wood is donated from a construction company where a relative of a staff member works. The wood-burning frames use moulding from the same company with some donated stain. Another project uses local driftwood sanded and stained. The occupational therapist found an old radio in response to a patient request.

Low-cost ventures that depend on scrounging may be highly rele-vant to the real lives of those with little money. Nevertheless, it seems clear that the official budgets and policies of mental health services make day programs operate creatively on a shoestring.

A third funding mechanism in six sites is revenue generation. Pro-grams make and sell handcrafts, small wood items, hand-made book bags, and other items, under controlled circumstances. For instance, Rosehill's policies concerning funding state:

Patients may be charged for materials used in therapeutic projects.

Partial hospital patients ... must be discouraged from raiding the depart-ment's supplies and encouraged to go into the community to make their own purchases.

Tools and equipment may not be sold to patients (this includes rug hooks, tape measure, needles, etc.).

Amount charged for articles is at the discretion of the staff member responsible for the patient concerned, or for making the sale, as appropriate.

Special funds for specific projects or programs may be set up from time to time, and sales are usually limited to recover only the price of supplies. There is often an administration-approved list that standardizes prices and restricts mental health day programs from competing with real community businesses.

If we look at the three funding mechanisms together (budget categories that include occupational therapy or activity supplies, petty cash, and revenue generation), we can see that they interact to determine what can be accomplished. The overall effect is that funding encourages simulation more than real-life education. Official budget funds cover the costs of real materials, local transportation, and participation in community events. Occupational therapists are usually the professionals who take responsibility for sustaining activity supplies, petty cash, and revenue generation. In fact, these unofficial funding mechanisms seem to constitute occupational therapists' unique stamp on programs.[4] They enable occupational therapists to operate a small-scale alternative to the main budgetary processes operated through mental health services.

Of course, these small funds are marginal to the official funding of mental health programs. Occupational therapy activities or supplies may be an official budget item, but they are considered a miscellaneous expense (and may be itemized as such in budgets). Petty cash is just that – petty amounts of money that can be used at the discretion of individual professionals. Revenue generation interacts with petty cash and is also peripheral to the primary funding processes organized through the official budget. Petty cash can be used to purchase materials and pay nominal labour rewards for revenue-generation projects that operate outside the budget process. But the funding of real occupational sessions and projects is miscellaneous, petty, or otherwise separate from the official financing in hospitals and in the provincial and federal government departments that fund mental health services.

Tracing connections between everyday program activities and organizational processes lets us see how educational sessions are shaped by space and time, which are in turn shaped by program philosophy and funding. Program philosophy and funding in mental health day programs emphasize simulation over real experiential learning. Neither philosophy nor funding act alone; they act in tandem. Program philosophy, in particular, produces variations in program content. The implementation of program philosophies is allocated to the professional team. Mental health professionals who favour simulation can draw heavily on psychoeducation. They can make little use of the three funding processes that support occupational sessions. At the other end of the spectrum, mental health professionals who favour critical reflection and experiential learning can draw heavily on psychosocial rehabilitation and occupational therapy. They can also make extensive use of a materials budget, petty cash, and revenue generation, even though these offer only minuscule funds.

The emphasis on standardization and simulation is not produced by face-to-face decision making but by connections between multiple organizational processes. As well, philosophy and funding are not the only processes organizing space and time. These intersect with assessment, admissions, case management, and hierarchical decision-making processes. Although they seem to have diverse purposes, in combination they support the emphasis on standardized simulations. Simulation is emphasized by conceptualizing and categorizing patients and cases rather than real people. And offering programs in standardized facilities and schedules makes it easier for programs to be accountable for the quality and efficiency of managing individual cases rather than the interconnected collective and individual actions of participants who are involved in real circumstances. Hierarchical decision making also perpetuates standardization and simulation; if those who use services are included in all decision making, they might want to change the philosophy, funding, space, and time frame so that programs address their real-life concerns.

Many mental health programs are moving out of hospitals and into real community situations, while also broadening schedules to educate people for living, working, and playing in real life. Nevertheless, they are still controlled largely by professional philosophies of helping, by hierarchically controlled funding processes, and by individualizing management information systems.

6

Risking Liability

Empowerment is a process of transformative change. Specifically, change is prompted through the participatory process of learning to critique and transform power. Participants engage in critique and transformation, changing not only their personal feelings, thoughts, and actions, but also the organization of major institutions in society. Such profound, transformative change is not without risks, especially since the process critiques and changes power in both the personal and social realms of life. When I recognized the magnitude of critique and transformation in empowerment, I decided to explore risk taking by asking how professionals support or limit risk taking by people who attend mental health day programs.

Enabling Risk Taking

Risk taking is necessary for real personal growth and social change. Furthermore, personal growth and social change are necessary to transform powerlessness into enlightenment, empowerment, and emancipation. Yet the critique and transformative action of empowerment involve people in multiple risks of changing themselves and society from *what is* to *what might be*. When professionals engage in empowerment education, risk taking is problematic for both the professionals and those who are learning to become empowered. Ideally, the responsibility for risk taking in empowerment education is shared by professionals and learners. The problem lies in determining whose judgment prevails in decision making, particularly where risks are high or, as with some who are admitted to mental health services, mental judgment is impaired, even temporarily.

It is difficult to decide how much risk is enough. Too much risk taking is overwhelming; too little risk taking results in too little change. To address this difficulty, people often need to be educated to share responsibility for deciding when, how, and how much to take risks. The implication of this comment takes us back to collaboration. People can be educated to share risk taking only when professionals recognize that they are not the only experts in deciding what risks people should take. Although day programs have not yet embraced empowerment education, let us look at three aspects of education in risk taking.

First, education in risk taking would challenge and guide people through the psychological and spiritual risks of perspective transformation, described by Mezirow and others as the process of changing feelings, beliefs, values, and sense of meaning in life. The psychological risks are those of accepting some personal responsibility for exercising power, including feelings of guilt, failure, power, and accomplishment. This means guiding people through anxiety, fear, excitement, and hope as they recognize that they are autonomous active agents with an internal locus of control. The spiritual risks are those of confronting beliefs about personal power and meaning in relation to a larger power. How frightening as well as exhilarating it can be to risk leaving protective, comfortable beliefs while trusting in the potential liberation of new beliefs. Education focused on psychological and spiritual transformation would prompt people to judge their readiness to take psychological and spiritual risks, then guide them as they explore new perspectives and beliefs that they judge to be right for them. The educational process would be one of collaborating with learners as they seek ways of generating inner control, courage, strength, faith, hope, and optimism. The educational goal would be to facilitate transformation in *feeling* and *thinking* about the self as a person who can change powerlessness into empowerment.

Second, education for risk taking would challenge and guide people through the risk taking required to transform everyday situations in which physical or mental competence are insufficient for people to live as they wish. We all face pivotal moments in which we need greater physical or mental competence to avoid being powerless, an experience common to those with defined areas of disability. Examples of such moments occur when individuals discover that they lack the knowledge and ability to find employment or to stop being abused. Education for this aspect of risk taking would challenge and guide people to risk going beyond their present competence to develop new physical and mental skills. The process would help people to decide what they want to do and what they need to learn. Education would then facilitate the development of competence in performance, problem-solving, decision-making, advocacy, or other skills. There would be graduated reflection and learning in increasingly complex, chaotic, unpredictable, and possibly physically unsafe, real-life situations. People would learn to risk failure and success in everyday actions. Real incidents and crises would be seized as opportunities to guide people not only to feel and think of themselves as empowered but to *act* empowered.

Third, education in risk taking would be oriented to organizational or systemic change. Here an educational program would involve both professionals and learners in looking at how an institution such as mental health services is organized. They would examine the potential for professionals and people to learn, in partnership, to share the responsibilities and consequences of risk taking. Each partner would face risks: people who are learning to share risk taking would face the responsibility of failure and success; and professionals would face the satisfaction of facilitating success, but also the legal liability for failures that result in harm. For all involved, there would be risk in 'rocking the boat.' Educating people to reorganize the processes of power, then, would involve all partners in taking the risks of trying out new responsibilities and liabilities. In substantive terms, people could learn how mental health services are organized by participating in that organization. Professionals would risk involving people as partners in situations that have traditionally been controlled by professionals; people who attend programs would take the risks of making decisions for themselves. The risk would be in transforming the hierarchical professional–patient relationship into a collaborating partnership. Unlikely as it may seem, professionals and those who use professionals' services would be called on to risk transforming the ruling apparatus.

A complication in risk taking is that professionals are responsible for protecting those who use their services. The complexity comes in deciding how to protect people from harm in risky situations. To address this complication, professionals and people who are learning to be partners would document their process of reasoning and decision making about risk taking. As well, risk taking would be identified as an explicit goal of empowerment education, with the rewards and consequences for each partner clearly identified. Moreover, liability statements would be developed in which professionals and learners are both legally responsible for the negative and positive consequences of risk taking. Legal support for shared risk taking would protect people's safety by requiring that risks be taken through step-by-step processes with just-right challenges, and with documented evidence that these steps have been negotiated. To make shared risk-taking a possibility, professionals would change their licensing and codes of ethics to spell out the legal boundaries of risk-taking partnerships.

Supporting Risk Taking for Transformative Change

Education in risk taking occurs in two aspects of mental health day programs. First, professionals guide and support those who risk attending stigmatized mental health programs, using potentially dangerous materials, and exposing their vulnerability in everyday situations. Second, professionals and the institution of mental health services make their support for risk taking public because the importance of taking some risk is highlighted in program materials, such as brochures.

The first aspect, guiding and supporting people to take risks, happens implicitly, rather than as a defined educational goal. Historically, people diagnosed with mental disorders have been negatively stigmatized. A diagnosis of mental disorder and an admission to mental health services have traditionally labelled people as members of a social group that is dependent on professionals and the state. Britte, who started a Friends of Schizophrenics group as an offshoot of her day program, describes the difficulty of getting past this stigma:

The biggest concern that people are expressing is the stigma – even just belonging to the group. Another fear they express is that their relatives or friends will know where they are going – and they won't like it.

Risk taking is also guided and supported as people use potentially dangerous equipment. Some mental health day programs have workshops with saws and other tools that can produce physical injuries if used haphazardly. In other words, people face pulmonary, cardiac, neurological, and other bodily risks in programs as they work around sawdust, glue fumes, and other chemicals used in various handcrafts and work projects. Program kitchens have knives, stoves, poisonous chemicals and other sources of potential physical harm. Occupational sessions (listed in figure 5.1) such as 'Maintenance' bring people into contact with paint, solvents, cleaning fluids, garden chemicals, and machinery for mowing lawns and blowing snow. Recreation sessions engage people in sports, where there are risks of falling, tearing ligaments, being hit by other players' rackets, and so on. In the occupational sessions that use equipment, then, professionals, often occupational therapists, educate people to control the physical risks of engaging in the material world.

To those of us who readily and unconsciously carry out life, engaging people in the minor risks of ordinary occupations may hardly seem like enabling risk taking, let alone enabling people to change their mental experiences of powerlessness. However, people who attend mental health programs are often feared as being dangerous. In reality, some of these people have actually harmed themselves. They may have harmed others before attendance in these programs or they may still be seen as potentially dangerous. As well, many people attending mental health day programs have long-standing, severe mental disorders. Some may have previously been removed from the material world by voluntary (occasionally involuntary) admission to a psychiatric unit, or occasionally to a forensic unit for those who have been charged with criminal behaviour. It is rare for people to be admitted to mental health day programs without a prior hospital admission for psychiatric treatment. In hospital, people may be rendered physically powerless if they only have access to the basic materials of life: food, beds, and occupations, such as cooking, that can be simulated in a hospital setting.

Mental health professionals also guide people to let their vulnerability be known in a safe place. The people who attend mental health day programs take the psychological and social risks of publicly exposing ideas and abilities that have already earned them the negative label of being mentally disordered. For some people, then, taking the risks of engaging in group discussions or meal preparation, even in program facilities, is an important and safe step in transforming their powerlessness.

People can sometimes be encouraged to take risks if they are given a 'gentle push,' as Rasha describes:

What I'm doing is giving them some guidelines, or facilitating them to solve their own problem. But it's sort of more with a gentle push, a sort of supportive pushing that we do here. We try to let them know that it isn't judgmental. It doesn't matter if they fail. But you better darn well get out and try it. That's what we don't like. It's not that you fail that we don't like. It's whether you try. We try to make it a really big gentle push! Being supportive, and being there for people certainly fosters dependence in some people, but hopefully we're alert to that in most cases. The real thing is to provide that support by saying 'What can you do about it?' 'How are you going to do it?' and 'I'll be here if that doesn't work. But you give that a try first' ... on the whole, even to get people to the point where they can say 'I'll try it on my own but I don't have to be alone if I fail.' I think that can be empowering. Just knowing there is somebody there can be empowering.

Rasha describes the program's safety net in which 'I'll be there if it doesn't work.' With her support, she urges people to develop the internal control, courage, strength, faith, hope, and optimism to 'try it on my own, but I don't have to be alone if I fail.' She also locates risk taking in the practical events of engaging in the everyday world.

The process enables people to risk releasing and pursuing dreams that, as Petra says, they may never have dared to consider:

Somebody will be able to identify something that has been missing. And they've never had an opportunity to try. Or they've never taken a risk to try. That might sound funny. But that is the case, quite often. And I think, as soon as I start having that conversation, I'm getting a bit of a handle on what they think of themselves, and what they've allowed themselves to do, and what they haven't.

Petra is referring to engaging people in handcrafts, which they may never have thought of as a source of meaningful satisfaction. She shows awareness that people need to develop a vision or a dream of what might be. Petra seems to be guiding people to take the risk of mapping out a transformative route for changing powerlessness through new types of thought and action. Her emphasis is on people transforming their perception that they lack power. As well, Petra guides people to risk developing their physical and mental competence as part of changing everyday life. In some instances, Petra, like other occupational therapists, may be challenging people to take the spiritual risks of contemplating new visions of life with new meanings, of risking a spiritual transformation.

In real-life situations, people are challenged and guided to risk having the courage and skills to try new experiences. Neva describes her support of Peter in volunteer work as a step toward possible employment:

We've been doing a lot of reinforcement for what he does – encouraging Peter to take risks – to go into new situations. He's really afraid to do anything like that. He has one of the most extreme problems in self-esteem that I think you might see. The surface looks great. So, we've been having a lot of major setbacks recently. They have a lot to do with me suggesting new volunteer placements. The thought of going into a new situation like that – just gets into depression and all kinds of things. Not much leeway for pushing. But at the same time Peter requires that. So there's a real fine balance to draw there.

Neva's interest in Peter seems to be psychological, but her approach to enabling risk taking is *occupational*, that is, based in what Peter *does*. She links Peter's 'problems in self-esteem' with her encouragement to 'take risks – to go into new situations.' She is supporting him to take the psychological risk of 'depression and all kinds of things' if his precarious self-esteem is not sufficient for the occupation of volunteering. She has located 'volunteer placements' that offer a just-right challenge without the excessive threat of failing at actual employment. In consulting with Peter, Neva encourages him to be a collaborating partner in deciding his own potential for risk taking and the conditions for taking the risks of trying volunteer work.

Jill's reference to an 'activity-based way' of helping people also highlights the issue of using 'your clinical judgment,' using language that turns the educational enterprise of facilitating just-right challenges into a therapeutic, medical discourse. As we saw in looking at the program curriculum in chapter 5, educational processes of critique and experiential learning are transformed into medical forms called 'psychoeducation' or 'psychosocial rehabilitation.' Here, Jill talks about the importance of people experiencing 'consequences' such as making a 'little fall':

Even if we let them make a bad decision – again, you have to use your clinical judgment – if it's a real rotten decision, you don't let them have a big fall over it. But if it's a little fall, sometimes it's best, obviously, to let them make that decision. Because, then, I think they realize that not only do they make the decision, but they have to take the consequences that come with it. And we don't take that [responsibility] either. I think the beauty of the whole idea of empowerment in occupational therapy in a facility like this is that we have a chance, in a very concrete, activity-based way, to reinforce it, and practise it all the time. You don't just talk about it. It's even to the point of – they say 'Jill, should I do this or this?' I say 'I don't know ... I'll explore it with you.' So I think we have opportunities for experimenting.

As Jill says, 'you don't just talk about it.' Implicitly, Jill highlights the importance of using everyday occupations as an educational opportunity for enabling risk taking, even if people only change their power to act in small aspects of life. Her response of 'I'll explore it *with* you' also suggests her attention to constructing people as active partners. Yet she also says that she might '*let* them make a bad decision,' indicating that she assumes her dominance as the responsible person in her relationship with those defined as patients.

Despite such contradictions, Brenda and Rasha talk about the program as a 'bridge' – the 'transition point' that Carol describes in chapter 5 'between being in hospital and being functional again in the community.' Brenda displays her trust that Rasha will guide her through the challenges and risks associated with her transition out of the hospital system and into a new life in the community:

Brenda   I really see this as a bridge between the hospital and being out on my own. In the hospital, you're nurtured and protected but in the program, as you say, you have to speak up for yourself.

Rasha   We try to make you responsible for yourself. We see ourselves as guides helping you to make some changes which you decide are important to you. There's a lot of hard work because no one can do it for you.

Brenda points to the usefulness of this bridge in enabling risk taking, where 'you have to speak up for yourself.' Then Rasha proceeds to indicate that she will support Brenda as a 'guide' while she risks doing the 'hard work [which] no one can do ... for you.' It is worth noting that guiding people to speak up for themselves may prompt considerable risk taking if they have not spoken up previously. Maybe Brenda is undergoing the personal transformation needed for her to make it over the bridge.

The second process that educates people for risk taking is located in program brochures, which challenge people to:

- live a healthy, productive life (Bayview)
- make changes you wish in your life (Clearcove)
- develop skills (Jackson Heights and New Garden)
- learn to cope with life problems in a constructive manner (Penrose)
- enhance functioning in this community (Rosehill)

These statements may not seem like much of a challenge to take risks. Besides, people who attend mental health day programs have rarely seen brochures before they agree to come. Nevertheless, people generally see these brochures once they start coming to programs, since they are posted on bulletin boards and in waiting areas.

Instead of accepting lives as patients who are hidden behind the closed doors of hospital wards or psychiatric offices, people are challenged to develop the courage and optimism to take risks; and, instead of focusing on their illness, they are prodded to 'live a healthy productive life,' 'make changes,' 'develop skills,' 'learn to cope,' and 'enhance functioning in the community.' People do not always arrive at programs with a vision of change. However, brochures convey a professional and institutional vision of what might be. They carry a vision and language of possibility. Through these documents, mental health services suggest that the future can be different from the past. They draw people into 'fighting for hope' (Kuyek, 1990).

Some people may be insulted because these descriptions imply that those admitted to day programs are unhealthy, lacking in skills, unable to cope, and dysfunctional. Others who are discouraged by their difficulties may see these brochure statements as an impossible dream. In any case, brochures challenge people to transform themselves and their communities. The challenge is to overcome stigmatization and fear so that those who have been excluded can be included in community life. Brochures encourage people to take the risks of attending programs, using program equipment, and participating in various parts of the program.

Managing Safety and Liability

On seeing some stated intentions and actual examples of risk taking, I wondered if risk taking is part of occupational therapy's discourse. I found that the emphasis was on guiding people to discover just-right challenges, with little mention of risk taking. Moreover, challenges were usually described in terms of adaptation: occupational therapists enable adaptation in individual performance far more than they enable social change.

Moreover, when I saw that risk taking was not an identified feature of occupational therapy, I began to trace the real instances of risk taking to policies and procedures, particularly risk management. The tension here is that challenges might be encouraged in small ways, but the official concern is with safety. Safety is an issue in part because some people have exhibited real danger to themselves or others. As Neva indicates:

The issues I've had with him are explosive behaviour at home, not here. Because he's so paranoid. And combined with that, he's got a really bad temper. He's dangerous ... hitting someone, he might strike out.

Some people in mental health day programs may be 'explosive' or 'strike out'; thus there is risk taking for both the professionals and those who use mental health services. In mental health programs of any kind, the consequences of risk taking may be high, as I noted after a conversation with Jill.

Jill commented on the magnitude of problems that occupational therapists are dealing with: that people are potentially suicidal or violent in numerous cases; that the style of interaction and way of working very much influences whether a situation will run smoothly or will blow up; that the occupational therapist is continually gathering information from observing people doing things, interviews, formal testing, meetings, and phone discussions with other professional workers, discussions in various contexts with family members, and so on. On the basis of that information, the occupational therapist processes the impressions and interpretation of the developmental issues facing that person. He or she then links those impressions with a judgment on the most appropriate activity to increase performance in work, self-care, and leisure.

Jill indicates the complexity of 'continually gathering information from observing people doing things' as an underpinning to the decisions made about the 'developmental issues facing' a person. Enabling such people to take risks, then, carries danger: too much risk may provoke severe consequences such as suicide or violence.

Britte's comments point to a related concern: that people have had frightening experiences and are afraid to risk 'losing control.' As Britte says, one woman

found group therapy going too fast and decided to stop attending ... she described fears about reliving past physical and sexual abuse ... she would rather repress feelings of anger and guilt than risk losing control should she discuss the past in a group ... she agreed to meet individually.

Some people limit their own risk taking. They are so afraid to face the pain of their powerlessness that they put up barriers to transformative change.

Mental health services manage the safety of these people through policies and procedures. For example, the sense of threat and need to control risk is visible in policies such as 'Bomb Threat.' The Penrose day program has a policy and procedure for responding to telephone and mail threats. A 'checklist' is provided to guide staff through 'Questions to be asked,' 'Description of voice,' and 'Background noise.' The clear message is that the staff member is to prolong the call long enough to gather information for police. Mental health programs are both the target of threat and the accomplices of police in controlling social violence. Policies that remind staff that they are potential targets of violence do not engender a spirit of adventure. They actually caution professionals against challenging people to change the organization of power in society. It seems that risk needs to be controlled to some degree if we are also to manage safety.

Less dramatic than bomb threat policies are the official documentary practices of risk management. Risk management is officially concerned with protecting safety rather than with enabling people to share responsibility for risk taking. The official management of risk requires professionals to create textual evidence of specific *incidents*

FIGURE 6.1
Categories of Risk Management Documentation (Rosehill)

Type of incident (including 'fall,' 'hazardous materials,' 'disturbance')

Person involved (patient, visitor, etc.)

• patient status (activity level and condition)

• type of injury (burn, strain)

• medication incident (incorrect drug, allergy, etc.)

• notification, as applicable (including options for in-charge person, next of kin, emergency, public relations)

• description of incident and action, follow-up, treatment, comments, physician comments

---

and *crises*. References to risk management here are focused on *patient* safety. However, the full policy, like most risk management policies, covers risk management for staff, volunteers, and any others who might be connected with the institution.

The evidence of incidents or crises is documented in an individual's health record. As an example, an incident report at Rosehill requires documentation under the categories listed in figure 6.1.

The incident report is completed by the staff person involved. There are strict guidelines about what is included and when an 'incident' should be reported. Rasha describes how some incidents do not actually qualify for documentation:

When I had two incidents in the space of a Monday to Friday, I was told they absolutely do not go on the chart ... in one situation, a patient took an overdose in the washroom. And one patient had a seizure – so they weren't cutting their fingers on our scissors or something like that.

Risk management policies and procedures, such as the one at Rosehill, attend to concerns for physical 'injury,' such as a burn or strain, or a 'medication incident.' However, risk management constrains more than physical risk taking. Physical or medication incidents may result from psychological or social risk taking when people act on their feelings of powerlessness, threat, fear, anger, loss of hope, and so on. The result is that risk management curtails the impetus to face challenges. Given requirements to document incidents, professionals are unlikely to provoke incident-type behaviour. They want to protect safety while avoiding documentation that might be interpreted later as malpractice on their part.

This brings us to professional and institutional liability. The documentation of incidents and crises is a professional responsibility. Professionals like Rasha are officially delegated responsibility for risk management on behalf of the institution.

Occupational therapists may be officially cautioned that their work involves interaction with potentially physically aggressive patients. Furthermore, they are responsible for the safety of all patients. In talking about taking a group out mackerel fishing, Britte displays this responsibility in ensuring that people have signed their legal consent to engage in a potentially risky occupational session: 'We get them to sign all kinds of consent forms and then we just go and hope no one falls overboard.'

Risk management policies and procedures create explicit documentary requirements for managing safety. Yet institutions control risk taking to a far greater extent than is apparent by looking only at the policies and procedures labelled as risk management. Mental health services have multiple, interconnected, hierarchical practices for managing safety by controlling risk.

To explain, people are active participants in their everyday lives. In mental health services, these same people are categorized as passive patients and cases. Patients and cases are not expected to be risk takers whose courage and competence might involve them in transforming society. The message in calling people patients and cases is that professionals are responsible for protecting them through a safe course towards mental health. Case management appears to be a separate process from risk management. Yet case management is individualized, thereby reducing the possibility of groups engaging in risky collective action. As we have seen, professionals are accountable primarily for individual case management.

Risk taking seems to be particularly controlled by the hierarchical decision-making structure of mental health services. Professionals, not those who attend programs, are responsible for managing risk. In addition, people attending these programs are not partners in documenting incidents or crises. In fact, people are legally prohibited from using their health records since they are the legal property of health institutions. While they can apply for access to their records, people are not legal partners in the ownership of their records. There also appear to be connections between risk management and the organization of space and time. Programs occur primarily in simulated conditions. The facility structures protected opportunities where safe risk taking is guided in empathetic, supportive conditions rather than in the potentially dangerous situations of real life.

We can now see how the work of enabling risk taking is indirectly as well as directly controlled by interconnected organizational processes. Safety is managed in many ways beyond the policy called 'risk management.' Professionals, not those attending programs, are officially responsible for managing safety, and, although this may sound preposterous, no one is officially responsible for enabling risk taking! Program brochures indicate that people are challenged to 'live a productive life,' 'develop skills,' or 'enhance functioning in the community,' but challenges are restricted to those that do not provoke incidents or crises. Should incidents and crises occur, professionals are personally responsible for documenting these events and for any failure to protect safety. Professionals must produce the official account of incidents and crises if they were unable to sufficiently protect people from harm. In other words, professionals document facts for use in their or the institution's legal defence if there is a charge of malpractice or negligence.

Furthermore, documentary practices of risk management reproduce hierarchical control rather than collaborative partnerships. Risk management turns professionals and people into legal adversaries, not partners. This hierarchical, adversarial relationship appears to be strengthened by professional legislation and codes of ethics. Occupational therapists, and likely other professionals, have no legal or ethical responsibility for enabling participation, or more particularly for enabling people to take the risks required to become empowered. On the contrary, professional legislation and codes of ethics refer only to professional responsibilities, and to the criteria and disciplinary action associated with malpractice or negligence. There are no requirements for professionals and those they serve to share legal responsibility for risk taking. In fact, even the idea of sharing legal responsibility seems like an abdication of professional responsibility, unless one shifts from a protective, caregiving stance to a trusting, empowerment stance.

Ultimately, risk taking is undermined by the objectified decision making used to determine liability in the modern practice of law. Legal decisions are not rendered by participants or witnesses of real events. They are rendered by judges whose decisions are based on documentary accounts. Individual health records that are produced by occupational therapists and other health professionals provide the documentation required for the adversarial system of law that prevails throughout much of the world.

Of course, liability claims that reach a court of law have financial implications. For professionals, the threat of liability claims has spawned a huge business in malpractice insurance. As an example, the Canadian Association of Occupational Therapists sells malpractice insurance through a national plan. Although employers such as hospitals provide general liability insurance coverage to therapists, an individual occupational therapist can still be charged if organizational processes for managing risk have not been followed. Concerns for legal claims are so great that health professional malpractice insurance fees are rising rapidly. The cost of increased insurance premiums is, of course, reflected in increased fees for medical and other health professional services. The climate of concern about legal challenges is so great that I carry malpractice insurance in case any academic or public statement, or any action, causes harm.

Looking broadly at risk management, it is clear that the whole institutional enterprise of mental health services manages safety, not risk taking. Rather than fostering a partnership that supports risk taking, mental health services manage safety through a hierarchical, adversarial relationship between professionals and the people who use professional services. Risk management is somewhat visible. One can read position statements that identify professional responsibility for protecting people's safety. One can also read policies and procedures for documenting incidents and crises. Then one can trace risk management policies and procedures to the processes of diagnosis, accountability, decision making, and funding, all of which manage risk in one way or another. The professional and financial consequences for losing claims of malpractice are very high. The effect is to make professionals cautious. In this context, professionals are more likely to subdue rather than encourage transformative change.

Certainly, the protection of safety is important. However, what is coming into view are the multiple, invisible processes that intersect to perpetuate professional dominance by overruling risk taking and transformative change. These are also the processes that orient practice more to the protective approaches of caregiving than to the risk-taking approaches required for enabling participation and empowerment. While we have seen instances in which professionals educate people to participate in collective and individual action, and in shared decision making, it is clear that caregiving dominates at least in part because it is physically safer. Caregiving is also safer for preserving the hierarchy of power, whereas participation enables people to change their lives and inevitably results in their wanting to share power. The ruling apparatus that manages risk not only protects individuals, but creates its impregnability, its resistance to transformation.

7

Promoting Marginal Inclusiveness

A host of stories, analyses, and statistics tell us that people with mental health problems are often excluded from ordinary employment, decent housing, and regular recreational and community events in modern Western society. Their exclusion points to the importance of promoting inclusiveness as a core feature of empowerment. Inclusiveness exists when all people are empowered *so that power and resources can be shared equitably*, when democracy and social justice are embedded in everyday life. At a certain point in my study I found myself asking, How inclusive are such processes as diagnosis, case management, decision making, education, and risk management, and how do mental health professionals promote inclusiveness in work, at play, and in general living?

Questions about inclusiveness did not occur to me until after I was well into the analysis. One of the foundations of occupational therapy that intrigues me is the profession's long-standing concern for the spirit. Concern for the spirit exists in a profession that works mostly with disadvantaged people, particularly those with disabilities or those who are experiencing aging problems or social crises. It seems to me that occupational therapy's attention to the spirit and worth of all people implies ethical support for an inclusive society with equitable opportunities for living in spite of mental health or other problems. I began to see how the practical work of mental health services shapes what professionals can do to promote a spirituality of inclusiveness, and thus the reality of social justice.

Social justice may seem like a long stretch for mental health day programs. Yet institutional ethnographies show how broad ideas such as social justice are (or are not) embedded in the practical organization of everyday life. Inclusiveness is made visible by the ways in which people are included or excluded in everyday situations. I looked at inclusiveness in mental health services in the everyday work of *chores, discharge, follow-up, sheltered employment, social recreation* and *special benefits*.

A Spirituality of Inclusiveness

As strange as it may sound, empowerment has a spiritual foundation that extends beyond spiritual transformation. By a *spiritual foundation*, I mean broad-reaching ethical ideas, not limited to religion, that guide everyday life. *Spirituality* refers to ideas and practices that extend beyond individual human thought and reason. The spiritual foundation of empowerment is an ethic of inclusiveness that is consistent with democracy and justice. Empowerment rests on an ethical belief in the equal worth of all people, an ethical commitment to enable all people to have equal opportunities for sharing the power and resources of a society.

A spirituality of inclusiveness offers mutual respect and support for the active power of each person. Practice based on this ethic openly speaks and acts against oppressive expressions of ridicule, disrespect, lack of empathy, stigmatization, disdain, mockery, callousness, self-righteousness, discrimination, unfairness, revenge, violence, or other acts of intimidation and subordination. Inclusiveness arises from a positive view of diversity as a source of enrichment for all of us, not as differences labelled as abnormal or deviant.

If we think about diagnosis, case management, decision making, education, and risk management – practices we have already examined – we can consider what they would look like if they were inclusive, if they fit an ideal vision of empowerment. At the outset, people would be categorized in ways that make them valued and included. Compassion, love, unconditional acceptance, respect, dignity, caring, joy, enjoyment, well-being, empathy, faith, peace, and other healing expressions would be embedded in the individual and collective actions of these programs. Both professionals and participants in their services would be included fully in the decisions made in managing cases, structuring programs, and determining the overall philosophy and funding for mental health services. Education programs would be designed to emphasize critique and to engage learners in risk taking and just-right challenges to transform real life in ways that improve their opportunities for being included in decent housing and employment.

We can also ask how case management might foster mutuality and interdependence. Diverse forms of expertise would be accorded value and viewed as useful in decision making. Of importance, community connectedness and sharing would be valued as much as the personal growth of individuals. An inclusive practice would support individual development, which would be balanced by supporting the development of self-help groups, community networks, mutual aid practices, and supportive institutional practices, with involvement in collective, social action as well as individualized approaches. Practice would openly celebrate the joy of community as a necessary underpinning to individual accomplishment. Ideas of individual liberty would be promoted alongside ideas about social responsibility to the communities in which people live.

And what about decision making? Collaborative decision making is an active demonstration of inclusiveness. Partnerships that are inclusive are characterized by horizontal collaboration. We have already seen how hierarchical decision making is exclusive rather than inclusive because hierarchy is reproduced in *differentiations of policy and decision-making capacities* (Smith, 1987). Professionals would demonstrate inclusive decision making if those they are helping were partners in making decisions about their own lives, programs, the organization of services, and even the terms and methods of professional practice. An inclusive practice, in essence, would turn hierarchy on its side.

Another feature to consider is the educational program. Education promotes inclusiveness when people learn to experience equality in real life. Empowerment education would both model and promote diversity over uniformity, flexibility over standardization. People would learn in places and times that are flexible and diverse enough to meet their differing needs. They would be guided and supported to take the risks of challenging exclusive, hierarchical practices. Learning would focus on organizing communities so that all persons are entitled to be included in work, play, and the other real situations that are meaningful to them. To accomplish empowerment education, then, funding would support a host of options that would promote inclusiveness, from simulation-based learning, to the transfer of this learning to real-life experiences.

To promote inclusiveness is to promote involvement over caregiving, and participation over charity and other forms of philanthropy. Philanthropy and charity are recognized as important values; but inclusiveness is about participating in life, not receiving hand-outs. For inclusiveness to occur, hierarchical approaches to philanthropy and charity would be replaced with social and economic practices that equalize opportunities for all people to be involved in giving as well as taking their share of resources, from food to employment.

Promoting Inclusiveness

I remember Brenda's first day. She came to the desk with the blankest face I've seen in a long time. Although she's no ball of fire yet, I see her reacting and interacting with other people. Her face has some expression. I think this lady is slowly coming alive. We lose sight of the differences in people when they are not obvious or major. But for her, after all these years of being essentially dead, I think she's slowly coming alive. And, for her, I suspect she's made huge steps.

Rasha's portrait of Brenda as a lost soul is fairly typical of people when they first arrive at mental health day programs. People like Brenda live marginalized lives, uncertain of themselves and stigmatized by others who question their entitlement to share the power and resources of society. Yet, over and over, in day-to-day interactions, I heard occupational therapists, and others, tell people that what they were doing was 'important' and will 'make a difference.' The occupational therapists publicly recognized the importance of ordinary daily tasks such as making a meal or answering a telephone. People were continually encouraged to help each other and to verbally acknowledge how each person is connected by the way in which he or she contributes as a member who is welcome in the group. As Neva says, these activities are organized so that people make 'natural and real connections':

The more they work side-by-side with each other, the more they make natural and real connections, the better they are.

Occupational therapists' conversations are peppered with comments like: 'am I ever glad to see you,' 'you have lots of good ideas,' 'I respect your judgment,' 'we need everyone to be part of the decision,' 'we really enjoy having you in the program,' 'you deserve a lot of credit for helping [yourself, others],' 'we will support what you believe is important to do,' and 'I have never been in your situation but it sounds extremely difficult and yet you have managed to keep going.' These statements look trite on paper, but I saw nothing to indicate they were not genuine.

From my standpoint observing everyday practice, it was clear that this work is not mechanistic or technical. Mental health services do more than treat the body with medication or apply behaviourial principles in standardized programs. The work is based on an ethical underpinning. Some aspects of everyday practice may seem mechanistic – guiding people to define behaviourial goals, encouraging people to talk and work together, facilitating role-plays of ordinary life situations – yet woven into mechanistic aspects is a strong ethical belief in the worth and power of the people who attend mental health day programs. Case management may be the official practice, but in reality I saw mental health professionals emphasize connectedness with others and the entitlement of people to be respected as fully participating members in all realms of community life.

To some extent, occupational therapists are fulfilling the institutional mandate to be supportive. As the program description at Penrose says:

The program approach is one of people helping people. Emphasis is placed on developing a supportive group setting that provides a sense of community while simultaneously giving individuals the flexibility to cope with their specific problems.

Occupational therapists are directed to develop a 'supportive group setting that provides a sense of community.' Certainly, such comments can easily become as rote and impersonal as 'Have a nice day' from a store clerk. Yet tone of voice, posture, attentiveness, soft touching, personalization of statements, and follow-up conversation, convey a genuine positive regard and respect for the people who attend mental health day programs.

Within programs, the sense of connectedness is fostered by the confidential information shared by group members. It is quite usual in these groups for people to acknowledge fears and failures and to risk trying new things in which they have no ready competence. People expose their vulnerability to group members. They do so in a place that treats such exposition as a positive step in healing.

I suspect that group planning for outings or other program events is an important process that enhances inclusiveness within programs. Through the practical work of planning these activities, people who tend to be excluded in ordinary society become involved in planning what they would like to do. Planning sessions seem to actively solicit participation, give people's actions meaning within the context of the group, celebrate the diversity of contributions from different people, connect people with one another, create an environment in which people have unquestioned membership rights, and create a forum in which everyone's ideas are included. Outings are also a practical method of inclusion. Even though they have been diagnosed with severe mental disorders, people go as ordinary citizens to businesses, places of interest, and recreational facilities. To an observer, the day-to-day work in mental health day programs looks inclusive, so I decided to examine inclusiveness in the organization of *chores*, *discharge*, and *follow-up*, especially the linking and advocacy that are part of the last two processes of case management.

Every program includes chores, often overseen by an occupational therapist. Chores involve tidying the program space at the end of each day, making coffee for program participants, posting pamphlets on employment or housing options, shopping for meal preparation, gathering information for outings, or watering plants. One of the key features is that chores set out responsibilities for the types of actions related to living as members of a home or place of employment. Of course, some people detest doing chores; others comment that chores feel artificial and demeaning. They say that they do not care if the plants in the facility live since they will only be there for a few weeks and they do not even like plants. These are valid objections. As well, chores can be questioned as being a management strategy for reducing the costs of the extra housekeeping services required because kitchen sinks need to be cleaned, sawdust from workshops needs sweeping, and so on.

As mundane as they seem, chores represent responsibilities that acknowledge the interconnectedness of people in making diverse but meaningful contributions toward a common goal. I watched some people positively glow when asked to do the shopping for the group's noon meal. Others reported with great pride at the daily check-in meeting that they had created a better system for cleaning bathrooms, keeping track of community events, or getting people to bring their coffee cups back to the kitchen after break. New Garden Clubhouse has made chores a significant part of its program. There are rotating unit supervisors and project titles such as Video Technician and Community Events Reporter that publicly acknowledge the worth and meaning of day-to-day chores.

Inclusiveness is also promoted in the work of linking and advocacy in discharge and follow-up, the last two processes in the sequence of case management. Discharge is the management process (sometimes called *separation*) used to officially complete health services; the purpose is to create a plan so that people know what to do and where to go after they leave programs. Follow-up is the related management process of checking what people are doing after their official discharge. In the programs studied, follow-up encompasses a variety of actions. Some follow-up is done by telephoning people to ask how they are doing. Other programs do follow-up by organizing individual or group meetings to check with people after their official discharge.

Two components of discharge, linking and advocacy, may appear to be ordinary common-sense types of work. Nevertheless, these are practical ways of promoting inclusiveness. This work consists of three fairly distinct parts. Linking begins by collecting community information. Occupational therapists are renowned for keeping files of resource information on recreation programs, employment possibilities, housing options, support groups, and professional services. There is more to this work than keeping files of names and addresses. Keeping files is the visible, technical result produced by analysing, selecting, and considering possibilities for adapting the occupations associated with each situation. Rasha points to this component of linking in describing how she gathers information on community resources:

If it's something that I want to go down and see how it's set up, I'll see if they can handle it either physically or emotionally. And, in some real specific way, I'll watch the task being done and see if I think they can handle it or whatever that might be.

A second part of linking involves ongoing assessment to determine when discharge is appropriate. As an example, Carol describes how, after using a 'leisure interest' questionnaire in assessment, she might suggest that ... the client or patient join some kind of group activity in the community. I may help them prepare their résumé, and role-play a job interview. Perhaps we talk about banking, grocery shopping. These things that occupational therapists do really fit nicely into supporting the person in their transitional stage back to a more independent lifestyle. Often I work with young people who are looking at making the transition from being quite dependent on parents or family, to getting their own apartment, or moving into a community residence. I might help them with things like meal planning, budgeting, things like that.

The ongoing assessment is about 'banking, grocery shopping ... supporting the person in their transitional stage back to a more independent lifestyle.' Carol is beyond gathering the initial, intake, screening, preliminary, or other assessment information needed to justify initial program admission. Her assessment in this circumstance is part of the process of linking people to community activities, a process of enhancing their inclusion in society. An ongoing assessment provides information for deciding whether people need to stay in or be discharged from programs. The questions underlying this assessment relate to people's ability to be included in the ordinary practices of banks, stores, and so on.

A third part of linking involves matching community resources with assessment information. Mai's work with a woman referred by her physician for 'simple stress management' demonstrates how the three parts of linking are interwoven. In this situation, Mai was promoting the woman's inclusion in a community from which she had withdrawn. Mai describes discovering the woman's home, marital, and parenting situation, where she was 'very perfectionistic.' She then encourages the woman to acknowledge her own needs and to ask her family to contribute to the housework so that she might be included once more in community life. In the end, the woman

did enlist her kids to help out more and she joined a health club and was going to go in swimming a couple of times a week – with her husband.

By integrating analyses of people's interests and abilities with various community resources, linking seeks to include people in employment, volunteer situations, housing options, self-help or community support groups, and various types of professional services. The work of linking conveys the message that people are worthy individuals who are entitled to decent housing, employment, and other community resources.

Linking is often accompanied by advocacy. As we have already seen in chapters 3 and 4, the occupational therapists are all in touch with local Canadian Mental Health Association (CMHA) committees, boards of directors of special recreation services, community groups sponsoring group homes, rape crisis support services, government task forces planning new employment programs, mental health self-help groups, and so on. The advocacy and lobbying, related often to discharge, are a way of promoting inclusiveness. These everyday practices are ethically based because they continually press organizations to include people with mental disorders.[1]

Preserving Exclusion

Although I have a very positive impression that mental health professionals do a lot to promote inclusiveness within day programs, I am acutely aware of the uphill battle that this feature of practice faces. Possibly, professionals are blinded to the positive atmosphere within programs; or perhaps hospital-based programs make community life invisible. Whatever happens, the disjuncture remains unconscious and largely invisible – the disjuncture of working in such warm, inclusive programs that only sporadically challenge the social exclusion and marginalization of people with mental health problems. Maybe the tension remains unconscious because, as Petra said in chapter 1, 'we offer a bridge in our transitional work.' If mental health day programs are the bridge, do professionals assume that they have no responsibility for promoting inclusiveness in the communities? But then, Britte pointed out the tension of working in a hospital-based site: 'I'm working in contradiction to some of my values and beliefs in what I could be doing to empower people. I work here because this is where I can get paid.' Although Britte is not referring to inclusiveness, she reminds us that, intentionally or not, we contain our work – and our concerns – to the places that are mandated by those who pay us. Then again, maybe professionals get caught up in knowing that mental health problems are themselves a barrier to inclusiveness. As an example, Neva describes one woman:

Her progress has been really slow because of her illness – cognitive deficits –

very hard. Every time we sit down to talk structured budgeting issues, her attention span is really negative for it.

In addition, limitations may lie in people's reliance on professional mental health services to such an extent that, as Britte says, people devalue or ignore nonprofessional programs. Instead, they expect that professional services will 'take care of me':

I find that patients have an excessive dependence on the [mental health services]. There's still that view that 'when I get sick, make me better. Don't tell me to change to promote my mental health. When I'm sick, take care of me.'

Britte's statement shows again how medical discourse dominates practice. People are defined as medical patients even when the concern is with their inclusion in community life. Moreover, patients do not always use nonprofessional support services that are open to them. As Petra observes:

There are actually recreation programs running [in this community] but people in this program generally don't tend to make use of them.

Petra faces the double difficulty of prompting people to seek inclusion while simultaneously creating openings where they will be included if they wish it.

To add to these struggles, professionals are primarily responsible for managing safe types of change in medically diagnosed patients. People are not even officially constructed as active participants. Nor are people partners with professionals except in deciding their personal goals. Since people retain the label 'patient' even in community life, they are cast as passive people whose diseases limit them from full inclusion in society. As we have seen, social action lies officially outside the mandated work of individual case management. As a result, discharge linking and advocacy count for very little in program statistics and are funded marginally through petty cash.

Moreover, risk management discourages professionals from collaborating with program participants in promoting community inclusiveness for fear of professional and institutional liability. Even if professionals attempt to break the cycle of dependence on mental health services, they face the constraints imposed by confidentiality legislation. As we saw in chapter 4, mental health services require official consent to make or receive telephone calls about a person attending a program. Signed consent is needed every time individuals are publicly named in a referral from mental health services. Even within programs, community linking and advocacy are difficult to organize. Professional and hospital legislation make individual practitioners cautious about working with people in the community because they are liable for risk management. Rasha's reply to Joanne, a woman attending Rosehill, illustrates this point. She cites legal restrictions as well as time limits in not continuing to work with Joanne, when she expresses fear at the prospect of losing program support:

[Rasha speaking to Joanne] You're certainly welcome to call if you need to but hospital policy says that we can't do follow-up. We are so busy on the one hand that we can't take on the follow-up. But the other thing is that the hospital requires us to have medical coverage. Now I can't imagine that there would be anything happening that you'd want to sue me for. But if anything happens while you're in the [program], I'm under the authority of the psychiatrist. But once you're discharged, then the psychiatrist does not have authority for that. And I can't work without that medical authority.

Even if risk and liability are minimal, professionals are too busy with individual case management to take time for many community visits. Certainly, occupational therapists make referrals to housing programs, employment projects, recreational activities, and support groups, where there is no medical involvement. When I asked Britte about doing more linking with the community, her answer was:

I guess the reason would be time. We don't have the staffing to do it. I think it would be very worthwhile. I have a strong belief that the community is where occupational therapy can be best put to use, where an occupational therapist's skills are best utilized.

No wonder that efforts to promote inclusiveness occur mainly inside the officially sanctioned structure in which professionals are accountable, funded, and protected. As a result, people are included mainly in an artificial mental health community.

It seems that inclusiveness is blocked by people's mental disorders and attitudes of dependence interacting with a host of processes that

FIGURE 7.1
Work Assessment Categories (Bayview)

Intellectual Considerations*	Physical Considerations	Emotional Considerations
Concentration	Manipulative ability	
Memory	Coordination	
Reasoning	Speed	
Judgment	Work tolerance	
	Quality of work	

*In the actual document, each of these category titles is followed by a set of questions and space for a summary. At the end of the document, 'Recommendations' and 'Work Area Suggested' are recorded.

protect both the ruling apparatus of mental health services and the exclusiveness of communities. We can go further with the analysis, and trace how inclusiveness is undermined by components of discharge that are related to linking and advocacy. Discharge and follow-up are supposed to disconnect people from their involvement in professional mental health services. There is potential at this point for people to free themselves of dependence on professionals. The problem is that the release of people from mental health day programs recategorizes (rediagnoses) them as mental patients who are then connected, through discharge referrals, with other mental health services.

Patients are recategorized, their final confirming diagnosis recorded as part of their send-off. Discharge summaries are constructed by psychiatrists from discharge interviews, as well as the psychiatric, occupational therapy and other 'Assessment' and 'Progress' notes that have been entered in health records throughout the process of case management. These notes are constructed mainly from interviews and simulation-based sessions, although some written references to meal preparation, clerical work, maintenance, brief writing, committee work, and public speaking may be present. Summaries are on professional forms, under categories that articulate professional ideas about what is important to document, as in the occupational therapy Work Assessment form displayed in figure 7.1. Such forms interpret real life as 'intellectual considerations,' 'physical considerations,' and 'emotional considerations' without reference to actual work abilities and potential. The information from a work assessment is of interest to occupational therapists who know what these categories mean. But recording information in this method is exclusionary. One requires professional training to understand it, making it inaccessible to those whom it describes.

Besides recategorizing people as mental patients, discharge perpetuates a *referral circle* that reconnects patients with other mental health services. Britte describes how this referral circle works:

People have been referred by professional services. So we don't feel that it's our role to cut them off from professional services. We feel that it's our role to refer them back to the referral source for follow-up. And if the referral source decides that they want to terminate professional services – if the patient is ready – then they can do it.

People are discharged from a mental health day program only to be referred back to the mental health professional (often a psychiatrist or psychologist) who made the original request for assessment and services, even if the referral was self-initiated, or made by a family member or another health professional. Whether or not people are referred to employment, recreation, financial support, or other community resources, they almost inevitably are referred to a psychiatrist, who will monitor medication or engage them in psychiatric counselling. The effect of this referral cycle is that people always remain psychiatric patients, moving from service to service within the mental health system.

Including people in artificial mental health communities and reconnecting them with other mental health services adds another interesting piece to the 'ideological circle' that locks some people into being mental health cases forever (Smith, 1990b, p. 44). Programs include only those diagnosed with mental disorders. Real experiences are turned into problems or diagnoses that are recognized in the *Diagnostic and Statistical Manual of Mental Disorders (DSM)*. Based on diagnostic facts, individual cases are guided to simulate the decision making and actions of everyday experiences removed from the risk taking of real-life circumstances. Discharge completes the circle of psychiatric case management, as Britte describes:

We're very much a goal-oriented program. So, from the very beginning, we're discharge planning. From the pre-admission interview, we're trying to establish a time line with these people on how long they want to come.

Admission goals are actually part of 'discharge planning,' which starts 'from the very beginning' after the 'pre-admission interview.' Each case is managed with an individual 'time line.' Official discharge then requires the completion of discharge/separation forms with a revised *DSM* discharge problem or diagnosis.

Since discharge and follow-up are processes within the sequence of case management, they are organized as accountable moments and facts. As we saw earlier, management is concerned with both quality and efficiency. Accountability practices, such as quality assurance, promote adherence to discharge procedures and documentation. As well, accountability for efficiency promotes discharge as early as possible so that the time and cost per case are minimized and the maximum number of cases can be managed. Follow-up is generally optional unless programs embark on evaluation research to study what happens to people after discharge. Once cases are discharged, follow-up is not officially monitored and so may not be part of the official account of caseload management. Discharge diagnoses confirm or revise the facts that justified admission.

Exclusion through Special Considerations

Of course, professionals can do little if the main options available on discharge from mental health day programs are out-patient or community mental health services. Otherwise people with severe, long-standing mental health problems tend to rely on *sheltered employment, social recreation,* and *special benefits*. We saw how budget categories, petty cash, and revenue-generation practices provide minuscule funds for educating people within mental health day programs. Unfortunately, communities have little more to offer, given the economic and welfare conditions of most societies. As a result, opportunities and funding for those with mental health problems are extremely limited. As Jill states:

The particular group of people we have at this time – poverty is a big one, not so much psychoses or thought process disorders. At other times in the program there have been people with major psychoses and so on, but many of the current people have emotional upheavals, life crises, events, difficulty interacting with others. Quite a number of people have had traumas in the past that have affected their relationships, their lives, so that they decide, for one reason or another, that they need to start dealing with them – get some support.

We don't just look at the client in the program. We're always looking at what other things are affecting their performance. So obviously, then, housing is always a big one. Because some of them, being out-patients, have some pretty poor boarding-houses. And they're not fed properly and they're cold as well.

Some people in these programs are struggling with problems of basic survival: housing, poor boarding-houses, being fed properly, being cold. They are living marginal lives of subsistence. Poverty is both a product of their marginalization and a constraint that perpetuates their marginalization; yet communities resist accepting these people as valued members. In Neva's words:

Their barriers are fitting into a society that's really geared to a high pace, and people who can function at a much higher level than they are capable of functioning. Our society is really a pretty stressful kind of society. And in most work situations, there's a certain level of productivity expected. There's a certain intolerance for any aberrant behaviours, intolerance for anybody that looks a bit different. There's a lot of stigmatization of anyone who's had a chronic mental illness. So they've got a lot of barriers to face.

Communities are 'geared to a high pace' with little interest in including people who are not already part of mainstream society. While professionals attempt to develop inclusive community practices, communities expect professionals to look after those whom communities are unprepared and unwilling to include. Community exclusiveness is particularly devastating for those who have experienced long periods of institutionalization. Britte notes:

We've done a disservice to these folks by discharging them from institutions to their home community. But their home community doesn't want them ... If you've had a fracture, you're expected to go back to work. But after you've had a depression or a psychotic episode, going back to work, or going back to your home just isn't the same.

People, professionals, governments, and communities all perpetuate exclusive practices that leave marginalized people in poverty. Mental health problems exclude people, especially if they have little money to participate in society. They form a marginal group in employment training, job creation, employment, and other economic practices through which they might work their way out of poverty.

The full results of limiting discharge and follow-up, then, are not only social exclusion, but also economic exclusion. Those with mental health problems are not welcome competitors for employment and associated economic advantages such as housing. In part, professionals who attempt to enable the economic inclusiveness of these people face resistant employers. Employers use mental illness as an excuse to exclude those unable to sustain standards set for economic productivity. In part, professionals find that employers and governments have a singular idea of productivity, with the result that part-time, shared, supportive, and other work arrangements are not widely available. If you have mental health problems, it is not easy to fit into existing jobs. As Jill explains:

For many of our people, 'work' as the general public would know – the 40-hour work week – for a lot of our people, that's not realistic. So when we do presentations here, instead of 'work,' we'll refer to 'productivity' and explain that it's not necessarily the five-day work week. But it's the idea of productivity ... the sense of accomplishment, self-esteem. Whether it be volunteer work, or working ... for an organization.

Jill takes a broad view of productivity, but most of the work allocated to people with mental disorders is sheltered employment or merely social recreation.

Sheltered employment offers people simulated work that is usually remunerated through incentive allowances, not real wages. As an example, Jackson Heights has a carpentry program in which people make lawn chairs, plant boxes, and so on for revenue generation. But the shop is not allowed to publicly advertise its business or its sales of goods because government policy forbids health and other services to compete with private business. Word of mouth is the only advertising possible. As a nonbusiness, the carpentry program is required to sell its goods at close to the cost of materials with a labour charge not to exceed the incentive wage of a few dollars a week. People cannot earn more because they are receiving the special benefits of social assistance. People are also paid below legislated minimum wages on the argument that this is therapy rather than employment.

The other classic sheltered employment projects are in the hospital industry: laundry, food services, and housekeeping. Once again, only special, token payment is offered for these jobs, identified as work therapy, in part, to satisfy union regulations. Work therapy jobs are too small or insignificant to undermine real, salaried (union) jobs. For instance, the student occupational therapist's manual at Jackson Heights describes hospital industry as:

a system of job stations through the hospital, the Community Care Centre, and the community. Individuals work alongside staff members or employees as helpers/apprentices, performing duties specific to the position as well as learning skills associated with the area of work. Examples of such positions are office helper, laundry aide, grounds maintenance worker, library assistant.

This analysis of sheltered employment offers us yet another view of the ideological circle of individual case management. Sheltered employment is part of the mental health community. It is an extension of mental health case management into ordinary life. Sheltered work processes reproduce dependence not as an intellectual attitude, but as an actual practice in actual conditions. Stereotypical, stigmatizing ideas about mental health cases remove these people from ordinary jobs. Mental health policies and union legislation limit the development of revenue-generation projects that might include people in real employment. Such policies and legislation reproduce a social hierarchy. People with mental health problems are relegated to low-paying or unpaid work and, thus, a low socioeconomic class. In other words, sheltered employment perpetuates exclusionary economic and welfare practices.

Stigmatizing ideas about mental illness underpin the creation of facts that are used to represent the employment potential of people who have mental difficulties. The facts assumed from sheltered or special projects are that people with mental health problems are only useful as low-paid lawn chair makers, office helpers, and laundry aides. Assumptions about employment are transformed into everyday practice through the actual work of developing job stations or other forms of sheltered work. Most sheltered work projects are extracted from actual jobs with little consequence to the economy of a society. Projects are developed by finding small business niches that are unproductive elements of the economy: hand-made lawn chairs at low cost, or industrial contracts completed at subsistence wages rather than the union wages that would be required if the work were included in the regular economy. These options are then simulated, often within artificial program conditions, to provide mental health cases with simulated employment experience. People gain experience in office help and other low-paid work, and then are slotted into similar low-paid types of employment in real life.

The alternative to sheltered employment is often social recreation. As Petra says, when people are not employed,

the program's response has been to provide social recreation programs which have been spearheaded by occupational therapy.

Occupational therapists are often encouraged to implement social recreation programs in order to keep people busy. Carol describes how she engages people in handcrafts as a form of social recreation that helps people to

develop some kinds of hobbies or leisure interests for lifestyle changes. If they've been depressed or in some kind of deprived environment or whatever, they haven't had a lot of opportunity to explore options.

I believe that Petra's involvement in social recreation and Carol's approach to lifestyle changes promote some degree of inclusiveness for some individuals. Some municipalities are now developing supportive recreation programs so that ordinary recreation includes a diversity of people using support systems such as 'buddy' programs. For instance, Carol makes referrals

to the city recreation department for more in-depth leisure counselling and leisure sampling. They have a sort of buddy program, so if somebody's anxious about going out into the community, that's an organization that will hook up a leisure buddy who will actually go with the person the first few times, until they're feeling comfortable.

It is worth noting that inclusive social recreation approaches, such as buddy programs for new, uncertain players, likely reduce some of the social stigmatization experienced by people with mental health problems. Other community members see and hear that these are people with feelings, ideas, and abilities.

A major problem is that social recreation and leisure are diversional. They occupy people, but divert attention from the struggle people have in finding a suitable employment niche. In shuffling people into social recreation, communities avoid finding innovative ways of including people with mental health problems as contributors to society and the economy. But discharging people to social recreation without employment is essentially sending them out to subsidized play while communities go about their real, economic business.

Ultimately, many people with serious mental difficulties depend on welfare. Since neither sheltered employment nor social recreation provides sufficient economic return for even subsistence living, people are offered special benefits. These are resources that are organized through state welfare and some voluntary organizations. Special benefits sought from voluntary organizations include special rates for membership at the YMCA/YWCA or low-cost social clubs for people who identify themselves as mental patients.

I watched occupational therapists, sometimes in connection with social workers and sometimes on their own, help people to apply for special benefits offered by the state. Here, mental health work connects with the legislated practices of state welfare. Welfare can provide special-needs funding through municipal or provincial social assistance programs. Those who receive special benefits may also receive special disability allowances that are usually higher than basic social assistance. Some people are eligible for disability pensions from private insurance companies. Others collect from former places of employment that offer disability severance packages as part of employee benefits. Special benefits often include pharmacare cards for free prescription drugs. While they are in programs, people can request bus tickets to the program or even monthly bus passes.

Sometimes professionals help people to find grants for special-interest groups. Or they work with people and various community workers to locate special funding for recreation, housing, and employment opportunities for minority or disadvantaged groups, such as people with mental, physical, or learning disabilities. Various municipal, provincial, and federal initiatives have provided special funding competitions for these groups. For those with special needs, it is easier to obtain these funds than mainstream recreation, housing, and employment.

Welfare practices promote a small degree of inclusiveness if only by preventing the total exclusion of some people who would otherwise live in abject destitution. Special benefits provide an infrastructure of financial resources that foster people's social inclusion within mental health programs and some community activities. It seems that people gain social inclusion at the price of economic exclusion from the payment that goes with real employment. Special benefits from the state parallel petty cash in mental health services. These are both token gestures that throw a few resources at those with mental health problems.

It seems that many people with long-term mental disorders are economically sustained through a network of sheltered work, social recreation, and special benefits. These economic benefits are conferred by both voluntary organizations and the state, and they perpetuate dependence because people are living a marginal existence. It is these real practices, not stigmatizing or discriminatory social attitudes alone, that undermine inclusiveness. Jill's experience highlights how people who receive welfare are excluded from real employment:

Probably the optimal goal for them now is work therapy, given the fact that any sort of competitive work or outside work is not only unrealistic but financially unreasonable. So for a lot of them the goal of work therapy is their 'work.' That's the top of the line.

Many people find that they lack the ability to participate in 'competitive work' or 'outside work.' In other words, economic practices extract the maximum capital from a full-time labour force. Those who require part-time or supportive arrangements are not sufficiently competitive since they increase the short-term costs of production. Sheltered work and special benefits perpetuate economic dependence because they discourage people from taking low-paying work. As I pointed out earlier, low-paying jobs are all that are expected by people with mental health problems. As Jill says:

We got Paul all lined up for the job and he went for the interviews and he got a job. But when he added up the money, he realized that he would actually lose out because he would lose his social assistance benefits. So he turned it down. He would be making less than he is now.

Paul is economically less marginalized on social assistance supplemented by special benefits than he is in regular employment. For him, employment is not a route out of poverty. He is relegated to poverty by his inability to find jobs that pay more than social assistance.

Ironically, sheltered work, special recreation, and special benefits limit inclusiveness while they simultaneously support the deinstitutionalization of people from mental asylums. On the one hand, sheltered employment and financial arrangements create positive opportunities for people to be included in communities. On the other hand, sheltered work, special recreation, and special benefits divert attention from the economic exclusion that people with longstanding mental difficulties continue to experience. People who have been discharged from mental institutions are welcomed as a new source of labour; but they are still labelled and marginalized as special, that is, inferior labour.

An ethic of philanthropy serves to soften the harsh competition of free-enterprise markets by emphasizing volunteer services and private acts of charity. Ideas of philanthropy also underpin the use of sheltered work, social recreation, and the special benefits provided as official state welfare. Unfortunately, philanthropy supports subsistence, from which there is no escape, even through employment. If we rely on philanthropy, we avoid granting universal entitlement for all people to share the power and economic resources of society. Instead, sheltered work, social recreation, and special benefits are offered as charity to keep people from starving. State philanthropy is hierarchically controlled, in part, by legislation that legitimizes these special approaches as part of a broad circle of mental health work and, in part, by economic and welfare practices that are officially sanctioned by the state. Charity is provided to indigent people who can never hope to share the power and resources of society.

In linking people to special services, professional mental health work constitutes what Paulo Freire (1985) calls a *domesticating practice* rather than a *liberating practice*. That is, mental health services domesticate people through sheltered employment, social recreation, and special benefits so that they do not challenge the unfair hierarchical economic order of a capitalist society. Mental health services support inclusiveness in mental health communities, possibly reducing the likelihood that people or professionals will challenge the exclusionary economics that prevail beyond program walls. Rather than liberating people to transform economic and welfare structures, mental health professionals inadvertently perpetuate people's dependence on these practices.

Discharge policies, accountability, funding, confidentiality legislation, professional referral legislation, and liability insurance legislation interconnect to invisibly undermine inclusiveness in community life. People may have lingering mental difficulties and dependence, but professionals also face liability legislation, caseload pressures, accountability statistics, and funding limits that reduce the incentive for community linking and advocacy. Discharge also feeds into a mental health referral circle. The result is that discharge extends dependence on professional services, even after people leave day programs.

This ruling apparatus is what Dorothy Smith (1990a) describes as impregnable. No individual or group of individuals within any particular government department or program is responsible for creating either the apparatus or its impregnability. Instead, government policies, budgets, and legislation restrict professionals from developing community services, housing, and businesses that might compete with those already funded by government. As Mai states:

If you're [a professional] looking for money, and you're advocating that the provincial government provide funding for new services ... I mean, that's not really done. Really. There's an unwritten law here. As a lay person one could advocate for these things. Do it on your own time. You're allowed to do whatever kind of volunteer work you want.

Governments are careful to avoid competing with private businesses because large private businesses actually dominate governments. Most readers will have seen reports of small businesses that have received government funding to include people with disabilities and that are then pressured to shut down under cries of preferential treatment when they compete well with the local business community.

In Atlantic Canada in the 1990s, economic conditions do not favour inclusiveness. Limited funds mean that there is little public space for professionals to promote an ethic of inclusiveness in job creation, housing, and all the other aspects of life. Jobs are scarce even for young, educated, white, middle-class males who, as a rule, are the most employable people in Canadian society. Those who can only manage part-time work or need special supervision have great difficulty competing. Recessions make people question state philanthropy (welfare, charity) and leave marginalized people to fend for themselves. Professionals may support inclusiveness philosophically, but, as Neva reflects, occupational therapy needs a 'radical shift' to match 'our philosophy':

Occupational therapists could use a little radical shift. We didn't start [mental health day] programs, even though it's all part of our philosophy. We're not at the leading edge of social advocacy or anything like that ... occupational therapists have adapted to quality assurance and all that kind of stuff. We're being socialized into working in the system and accepting that.

A market ethic limits inclusiveness by limiting universalizing government initiatives. Governments are needed to equalize employment and other opportunities for disadvantaged people such as those with mental health problems. Institutional ethnographies, such as this one, would likely show how housing, employment, education, social welfare, banking, and business in Western society are all ruled by a market ethic that prevails over an ethic of inclusiveness. One might say that a market ethic overrules a spiritual ethic of inclusiveness by sustaining a form of apartheid: jobs are segregated so that only marginal ones are left to those with mental health problems.

8

Challenging the Routine Organization of Power

We have seen how everyday activities, from assessment to the use of petty cash, are acts of power. We have also seen how good intentions and real instances of empowerment are overruled: what seems like empowerment is narrowed, undermined, or otherwise distorted by anonymous but interconnected, routine organizational processes that govern what can and cannot be done. In mental health services, such processes overrule real attempts by mental health professionals to promote the empowerment of those who use mental health services. These people are transformed into medical objects, who are managed so that decision making and potentially transformative action are contained. Moreover, social action is accounted for mainly in terms of the individual goals that can be realized through simulated programs in singular locations during daytime hours. Professionals who try to involve people in empowerment experience tension: participation is undermined by the objectifying processes of assessment, diagnosis, and admission; collective action is narrowed by the individualization of case management; collaboration is restricted by hierarchical decision making; learning is concerned more with simulations than real life; risk taking is turned into safety management; and the development of an inclusive community is confined within programs. These tensions are not experienced as such; rather, professionals who attempt to promote empowerment tend to feel overwhelmed, inadequate, or not fitting into the system.

Building on the analysis already presented, this final chapter takes a broad view of the tension in professional mental health practice. An outline of present challenges to discover the underlying tension between empowerment and dependence leads to a proposal about future challenges to change the routine organization of power. I will conclude with comments on the critical perspective of this book.

Present Challenges: Discovering the Disjuncture

The present challenges are those undertaken in this book: to uncover the disjuncture, the bifurcation of consciousness that produces experiences of tension for mental health professionals such as occupational therapists. On discovering contradictions *within* six features of occupational therapy, I decided to look *across* these features at the overall organization of power in mental health services. From this perspective, I found two divergent profiles: one promoting empowerment, the other dependence. Herein lies the disjuncture: a fundamental contradiction between divergent ways of routinely organizing power. Attempts to promote empowerment in mental health services are struggling against routine official practices that promote dependence; laudable initiatives for enabling participation are out of step with official routines of caregiving. This contradictory organization of power is so embedded and invisible that it is experienced as taken-for-granted routines that seem natural and unquestionable, and so interconnected and impregnable that professionals who enable participation merely feel different from other professionals.

The following Profile of Empowerment draws together the positive elements of the features examined previously. The contradiction becomes visible when the routine processes for ruling mental health services are drawn together, producing a Profile of Dependence.

A Profile of Empowerment: Enabling Participation

A 'Profile of Empowerment' (figure 8.1) is not a technique, model, theory, or vision. Rather, it captures participatory processes of learning to critique and transform feelings, thoughts, and actions, as well as the organization of society, so that power and resources can be shared equitably.

Features in the Profile of Empowerment are presented as they were discovered. They are not linear or sequential in time, but, rather, synchronous, each strengthening the other as they interconnect. 'Inviting Participation' appears first because this feature was investigated in relation to naming and organizing mental problems, one of the initial management processes that people encounter as they

FIGURE 8.1
A Profile of Empowerment: Enabling Participation

• Inviting Participation

• Facilitating Individual and Social Action

• Encouraging Collaborative Decision Making

• Guiding Critical Reflection and Experiential Learning

• Supporting Risk Taking for Transformative Change

• Promoting Inclusiveness

---

enter the world of mental health day programs. Participation could easily have appeared last on the list if I had chosen to explore people's participation in organizing their work and home life so that they will be supported when they stop attending mental health services. Positive instances in which professionals enable others to participate in their empowerment are not necessarily haphazard or isolated acts. In occupational therapy, for instance, such acts occur consistently and, as we can now see, form a profile of interconnected and ongoing processes in a method of organization. The seven occupational therapists illustrate localized, practical ways of involving people with mental health problems in their own empowerment, despite overruling barriers. Their localized empowerment approaches disrupt the routine organization of power by reducing hierarchical control within specific programs.

Inviting Participation
Participation is a cornerstone of empowerment, the starting point for involving people in helping themselves. It seems like common sense to invite people to participate, but it is radical to assume that people can participate if, historically, they have been cast in the passive role of patient. In practical terms, participation is invited by guiding people to discover their individual talents, and by creating opportunities for participation in organizing as well as carrying out activities. This comes, in part, from identifying participants' active power in titles such as member, learner, or advocate, and, in part, from publicly guaranteeing entitlement to participate.

In mental health day programs, participation is invited by recognizing people as active agents, that is, as members or persons rather than patients. Work clothes, equipment, schedules, and facilities publicly declare that participation is expected. Actual participation occurs in programs that involve people in cooking, recreation, and in-house employment. In assessment and admission processes, people are asked to participate in defining their strengths and difficulties, drawing on their subjective expertise in knowing themselves and their situations. Increasingly, participants' views are being officially documented in health records, such as in the *Members' Notes* in psychosocial rehabilitation programs. Some official entitlement to participate appears in program brochures, which invite people to become involved in helping themselves rather than wait to be cured by professionals.

Facilitating Individual and Social Action

Empowerment requires participation in both individual and collective action. As people transform their personal perspective on power and learn to act with greater assertiveness, they gain confidence and experience for acting collectively; conversely, collective action reduces fears of acting alone, thereby building confidence and a personal sense of power. Participants are both autonomous actors and interdependent members of groups and communities. Interdependence is brought into reality when participants are encouraged to take responsibility for themselves in individual and collective action, and when institutions are organized to work with groups as well as individuals.

While being highly individualized, mental health day programs involve people in the collective action of organizing and running daily activities. Individual case management includes group sessions. Participants in some programs band together to write letters and speak publicly in advocacy for housing, employment, social assistance, and other opportunities. In some mental health settings, position descriptions and workload measurement criteria officially recognize collective action.

Encouraging Collaborative Decision Making

Basic to empowerment are processes of collaboration, played out in horizontal rather than hierarchical relations. Collaboration occurs in 'teams' that involve all those affected by decisions about individuals and groups, professionals and managers. Empowerment surges when collaborative decision making occurs, not only in everyday situations, but in the organization of program structure, documentation, legislation, and financing. In collaborative partnerships, those seeking services are recognized as experts along with professionals and managers. Each educates other partners to understand different forms of expertise so that decisions are informed by many perspectives. Moreover, every team member has an equal voice, and diverse views are respected and debated freely. Such freedom to debate and decide how life will be organized arises from a generosity of spirit, but often needs legislative support, particularly if decisions touch on strongly held beliefs or cultural ideas of privilege.

Collaborative decision making is a reality in mental health day programs to the extent that people with a long history of dependence on professional decision making are invited to be partners in defining their personal goals and in coordinating their cases. Choices about how and how much to participate in programs are made by participants in consultation with professionals. In many instances, people are asked to collaborate in making decisions about program activities and schedules and in rating their satisfaction with programs. Collaborative decision making is increasing as *consumers*, meaning those who have used (consumed) mental health services, are included on provincial committees, boards of directors, and other bodies that govern mental health services.

Guiding Critical Reflection and Experiential Learning
Processes of empowerment are learned; thus, education can foster or limit empowerment. Empowerment education prompts people to engage in critical reflection so that they become aware of power in their lives; experiential learning involves participants in transforming oppressive and otherwise disempowering features of real life. Through critical reflection, people become conscious of their power to express their desires and talents while also learning how their experiences of power in everyday life are governed. Learners participate in developing the knowledge and skills they need not only for personal development, but also for creating a just society. Standardized simulation and codified exercises in fixed places and times are useful as a starting point for learning without distractions and barriers. To be relevant and responsive, however, empowerment education is flexible rather than standardized, and goes beyond

simulations to address real individual and group needs in everyday places and at times in which empowerment is sought. Besides learning to organize daily life, participants learn to determine the schedules, facilities, philosophies, documentation, information management, funding, policies, and legislation needed to support their empowerment. In turn, policy, legislative, and financial support make empowerment education possible.

Aspects of empowerment education are illustrated in the interactional and occupational sessions of mental health day programs. Simulation exercises, such as role-plays, are commonly used in stress management and assertiveness groups. Some individual and group sessions prompt reflection on personal experiences of power. Opportunities for experiential learning exist where programs include cooking, clerical work, maintenance, advocacy, community volunteering, and social outings. Education for living occurs, at times, in people's homes, in workplaces, and at local recreation facilities. Some philosophical and financial support for empowerment education is demonstrated when mental health facilities have kitchens, living rooms, and work areas. The commitment to empowerment education in day programs is striking when one considers that these spaces are organized and funded by hospitals that are otherwise oriented to medical equipment and treatments. Some flexible, diverse learning experiences are supported by petty cash and small revenue-generation projects.

Supporting Risk Taking for Transformative Change

Risk taking is necessary to transform *what is* to empowerment. Only through risking unknown challenges do people learn to change their experience, or to shift the organization of power. It follows that empowerment requires participation in risk taking in the process of transformation. People are challenged to risk new ways of feeling and thinking about their lives. Empowerment challenges people to act differently and face new risks in everyday situations, as well as to risk challenging professionals and managers; in turn, professionals and managers are challenged to forgo elite privileges and to experience the power of sharing. Ideally, all partners share the official responsibility and liability for supporting risk taking, while also protecting everyone from unsafe or overwhelming risk. Definitions of unsafe or overwhelming risks are created by all partners, not only by professionals, managers, or lawyers. The ideal is that partners determine appropriate risk management policies and liability legislation.

We can see a degree of risk taking at work in mental health services. There is graduated support for risk taking by people with a history of anger, violence, mood swings, or other problems of mental control. Physical risk taking is guided as people use potentially dangerous equipment and materials in kitchens, cleaning areas, and maintenance shops. In individual and group discussions, people are encouraged to face the psychological and spiritual risks of exposing their individual powerlessness. Besides, people are asked to gauge their own readiness for risk taking. Risk taking is officially recognized in program descriptions that invite people to take responsibility for making changes while daring them to develop a future that is different from the past.

Promoting Inclusiveness
Inclusiveness underpins empowerment in that empowerment includes all people as worthy citizens who share power and resources. Those who are marginalized gain legitimate and equal access to housing, work, recreation, money, and other social benefits. Rather than excluding – that is, segregating – those who are different, an inclusive community celebrates the involvement of diverse people and their contributions to the community without pitting community against community, clan against clan. Empowerment advances when quality of life is not the privilege of an elite group that generates personal wealth while others languish. In everyday situations, all relevant persons are included in all areas of decision making. Connectedness and belonging are promoted by constantly highlighting the value of all participants and all contributions as part of an interdependent process of living. Universal access and opportunity are routinely guaranteed in policies, legislation, and funding that create democratic processes of governance.

Mental health day programs create inclusive communities for those who participate. Compliments on dress, talents, and contributions to programs, and on the overall value of everyone's participation are emphasized to invite people into involvement and to make sure people feel appreciated. The group honours participation without comparing the quality or quantity of work done. Highlighted regularly are special events, such as birthdays, and special talents that include people in some way, whether in music, computer operation, or answering the telephone. Chores are used to connect people in mutual helping and giving relations. Individual and group advocacy

FIGURE 8.2
A Profile of Dependence: Caregiving

• Objectifying Cases

• Accounting for Individual Cases

• Controlling Decisions Hierarchically

• Educating through Standardized Simulations

• Managing Safety and Liability

• Preserving Exclusion

---

help participants to find housing, partial employment, and recreation opportunities in their communities.

A Profile of Dependence: Caregiving

In spite of good intentions, attempts to promote empowerment are overruled by routine organizational processes that, listed together, form a Profile of Dependence. The list is ordered to reflect both the sequence of my investigation and the Profile of Empowerment. The Profile of Dependence consists of everyday processes of caregiving that, although well intended, nevertheless objectify, protect, or otherwise overrule participation (figure 8.2).

Like empowerment, dependence is not produced through a single process or technique. Each process seems rather innocuous in itself. Many would claim that processes of caregiving are not meant to make people dependent, but, rather, are expressions of kindness, respect, and duty in caring for each other. Moreover, in many individual situations, people and professionals have triumphed over or circumvented dependency-producing processes. Sometimes we minimize the features in this profile. Does it really matter whether we call people patients or members? Are statistics, policies, and other kinds of documentation important, compared with our actual work? We tend to think of *the system* as an external force rather than as something embedded in our everyday experience, so we assume that paper work, policies, and budgets are merely nuisances. Moreover, there is a sense that one does not always need to go along with the system, or that one can get around the system.

Certainly, professionals are not overtly taught to dominate people, to be so individualized as to ignore social conditions, to overprotect people from risk, or to practise exclusionary discrimination. One does not find many professionals who consciously and openly set out to undermine participation or produce dependence. On the contrary, participation, interdependence, collaboration, critical reflection, risk taking, and inclusiveness are the language of avant-garde professionals and organizations, who stress the economic advantages of empowerment. Many point to the savings that would come from people taking more personal responsibility and reducing their dependence on professionals. No overt force, coercion, confinement, or other external method is needed to control people. Instead, dependence, like empowerment, is a method of organization. Moreover, this is the taken-for-granted, routine method of organizing power in mental health services. We assume, unconsciously, that a dependency-producing method of organization is natural and necessary, its processes objective and fair. Viewed separately, the processes may be fairly administered, but this does not negate that they are ideologically biased so that power is controlled in particular ways by particular people. Rather than sharing power as in empowerment, patients are controlled by others who, in their good intentions, assume to know best. In summary, dependence works by objectifying, individualizing, and protecting people in ways that undermine their power to participate. Documented facts about individual cases are then used to demonstrate accountability and justify programs. Dependence prevails as long as privilege, individualism, protectionism, philanthropy, and bottom-line economic accountability dominate the routine organization of power.

Objectifying Cases

Cases are created by a process known as objectification, in which (active) people are transformed into (passive) objects known as cases. Instead of being recognized as participants, people are objectified when their strengths and problems are slotted into categories such as schizophrenia. Individual cases depend on expert decision making for access to services; people's subjective knowledge is insufficient or irrelevant. Control over defining needs, strengths, problems, and solutions rests with experts.

The key organizational processes used to objectify cases in mental health services are assessment and admission. Cases are objectified as patients and categorized according to psychiatric diagnoses.

Admission to mental health services is restricted to those cases that are assessed to have symptoms matching a diagnostic category. The process of diagnosis is hierarchical because mental health professionals hold the power to confirm diagnoses, while patients/cases are dependent on being diagnosed. Objectification gives control of mental health cases to psychiatrists, who are responsible for making and recording a diagnosis in an official assessment summary. Psychiatric control over objectification is mandated by professional, provincial, and federal regulations that grant funding to provide mental health services only to cases that have been psychiatrically diagnosed.

Accounting for Individual Cases
The creation of individual cases forms a foundation for accounting for individuals through the process of individual case management. Individual cases are managed through objectified management processes. Objectified management refers to the control of cases through documentation rather than through knowledge gained by face-to-face interaction. Knowledge about individual cases is produced by fitting all the details, interpretations, and other knowledge about people in actual situations into the categories deemed relevant for organizational decision making: diagnoses, problems, goals, plans, services, discharge, and outcomes identified through follow-up. Documentation of individual case management is then used to demonstrate accountability in terms of individual cases.

Objectified management is designed to remove partisanship and bias, and to create efficiencies in decision making, yet the information used in objectified management is necessarily partisan. Objectified decision making is based on partial knowledge, since certain facts are selected and others dismissed as irrelevant for documentation. The categories for documentation have been selected by experts who have particular ideas about what is important and not important to know. Documented information may be defined as relevant from an institutional perspective even if the people who seek services consider other information to be equally or more relevant. Individualized case management makes information relevant only if it can be related to individual cases. Therefore, information about the structure or organization of society can only be made accountable in terms of individual cases.

In mental health services, the integrated process of facilitating individual and collective action is overruled by official requirements for managing and accounting for individual cases. Ideas about individual independence locate the responsibility for action in individuals. Individual cases are managed through the organizational processes of individual goal setting and case coordination as follows: from the lived reality of their holistic, contextual lives, people (cases) identify problems and goals for individual action, which is managed by documenting progress on these goals; documented facts about individual problems, goals, and action are used to account for the quality of individual case management. Furthermore, facts about the numbers of individual cases and aggregates of individual cases – that is, caseloads – are entered into a Management Information System (MIS); MIS facts on cases and caseloads are analysed to account for the efficiency of individual case management; MIS documents are audited through the quality management programs used to uphold national hospital accreditation standards; accountability for the efficiency of individual case management determines program funding since federal government transfers to provincial government health budgets are calculated on past and projected costs per patient/case managed per month and year. Congruent with individual case management are individualized decision making, education, risk taking, discharge, and follow-up. There is no similar process for making mental health professionals accountable for facilitating collective action.

Controlling Decisions Hierarchically

The work of creating and managing individual cases is governed by a hierarchy that is particularly visible in processes of decision making that coordinate and control the management of cases. At the top of the hierarchy, those who govern decide which work is relevant to that institution and which facts are required to make this work accountable. Workers at various middle levels of the hierarchy are allocated the actual work of the institution. These same workers interpret and select facts that will be used to account for the quality and efficiency of their work. Based on these documented facts, those who govern the institution make decisions about the ongoing relevance of each type of work. Those who govern also create a record of their decision making in a variety of documentary forms, including policies, procedures, budgets and legislation. Governing is done anonymously through position descriptions that require middle-level workers to comply with institutional policies, procedures, budgets, and legislation.

The experiences of occupational therapists illustrate how horizontal collaboration is contained by the hierarchical decision-making structure of mental health services. Mental health services have turned to individual case management, in which cases are allocated individual responsibility for making decisions about their personal goals and the actions they will take to reach those goals. Participation in these individualized processes does not make patients/cases equal decision-making partners in controlling mental health services. Furthermore, professionals are accountable for the work of managing the decision making of patients/cases and for documenting decisions in individual health records and the MIS. The efficiency and effectiveness of professional work is judged by using the facts about individual cases that professionals have decided are relevant to record for the management of mental health services. Expectations that professionals will comply with mental health policies, procedures, and legislation are embedded in position descriptions. Hierarchical control of mental health services is sustained by professionals and managers who have decided that patients/cases cannot be efficient or trusted decision-making partners because they are not sufficiently familiar with the system of managing caseloads and confidentiality. To reinforce this hierarchical control, confidentiality legislation discourages professionals from involving patients/cases in program and institutional decision making. Professionals can only work in partnership with people who have explicitly given written consent to be publicly associated with mental health services.

Educating through Standardized Simulations
The objectified processes that create and control individual cases shape possibilities for education; education is structured to produce the types of facts that are relevant to the objectified management of individual cases. This type of education transforms real experience into problems, goals, and objectives, defined as observable behaviours that can be documented in professional terminology and measured to determine change; simulated versions of real experience are then organized into an educational curriculum in which the transfer of learning to real life is omitted. Facts divined about learners from simulations are then extracted to fit the documents that are used to audit the quality and quantity of education and learning. Learners, in essence, are educated to interpret their lives with reference to the needs and solutions defined by educational experts. The lesson is that real life experiences are largely irrelevant unless they are framed in ways that are relevant to the education provided by particular institutions.

A typical set of objects (problems, goals, objectives) is used to justify the development of standardized programs and services. Standardization is emphasized, in the name of efficiency, by using a single location, schedule, and standard set of activities. Removed from real situations, people learn to address their difficulties and needs primarily through simulation exercises and experiences that can be organized within a singular setting. Program philosophies, locations, materials, and time frames are organized to support standardized, professionalized approaches.

It is true that the patients/cases in adult mental health day programs participate in real experiences, such as cooking and maintenance. In psychoeducation programs, however, the philosophy and funding support mainly simulation activities, such as role-plays and discussions, primarily within the simulated space and five-day-a-week time conditions of programs. The philosophy and funding of psychosocial rehabilitation programs do support members in learning through real experiences, but standard program facilities and time schedules are still the mainstay. Regardless of program philosophy, official budgets typically include only small amounts of funding for program equipment, materials, and supplies. Transportation and expenses for working in community situations are rarely covered for more than sporadic occasions. Even when professionals, such as occupational therapists, want to work in real situations, day program caseloads and schedules are usually organized around individual and group sessions inside facilities. Petty cash and revenue generation provide some funding flexibility, but these are small adjuncts to the official budget process.

Managing Safety and Liability

The program philosophies and funding processes that emphasize simulation are connected with the management of risk and liability. Risk is explicitly controlled through documentary processes called risk management. Risk management is defined in policies and position descriptions that officially declare an institution's responsibility for protecting the safety of those who use the services of that institution. Policies also define the types of incidents and crises that require documentation. Documents create legal evidence that can be presented as the professional and institutional defence against a claim of negligence or malpractice.

Besides the overt practice of risk management, risk is also managed indirectly and implicitly. The process of creating and managing individual cases reduces risk by keeping the focus on individuals rather than encouraging collective action that might challenge existing professional and institutional practices. Risk is further controlled by managing cases largely within the physical and social safety of simulated program conditions. These and other intersecting processes orient an institution more to protection than risk taking.

With a growing threat of potential liability suits, mental health professionals are encouraged directly and indirectly to work in safe activities and situations. Risk is managed directly by allocating responsibility to professionals for documenting incidents and crises in the same health records that are used to account for the quality of practice; in addition, risk taking is indirectly overruled by policies and legislation that make professionals and institutions liable for protecting the safety of patients/cases. No policies or legislation hold professionals responsible for supporting risk taking. And no legislation exists to make patients/cases legal partners, instead of legal objects that are adversaries in the management of risk. The emphasis in mental health services is on managing individual cases in the safety of simulated conditions where risk is minimized.

Preserving Exclusion
Exclusion is a socially organized practice that operates by granting privilege and special opportunity to those whom a society views as knowing best or as deserving better than others. Privilege is offered by granting office space, library access, or paid continuing education to some, but not others. In other situations, differential entitlement (sometimes called systemic discrimination) operates by granting certain people special opportunities for decision making and access to resources such as housing, employment, or financial rewards. Another mechanism that preserves exclusion is classification, a means of categorizing the power each group holds within a hierarchy. In other words, hierarchical decision making is also part of the practice of exclusion. While people may participate at some levels, they are excluded from the top levels of decision making that are reserved for professionals, managers, politicians, and corporate executives. Exclusion is also preserved by philanthropy, whether philanthropy be practised by individuals, groups, or the state. Philanthropy is based on caring for people, who are then dependent on good will and charity. Whether in the form of charity or social welfare, philanthropy makes

people dependent on them as caregivers. It also avoids addressing underlying inequities in the structure and organization of society.

Beyond the face-to-face relations that are developed in mental health day programs, people with long-standing mental health problems continue to be marginalized in society, officially labelled as psychiatric patients even out-side programs. Many of those who have been long diagnosed with mental disorders are subjected to a double exclusion, a no-win life: de-institutionalization excludes them from hospitals, while they remain excluded from jobs, decent housing, recreation, and other ordinary resources in communities. Certainly we cannot lay the full blame on mental health services for the social exclusion of people who have been 'psychiatric patients.' Two processes, assessment and admission, require people to be officially classified as 'psychiatric patients' as long as they are associated with mental health services; two other processes, discharge and follow-up, create a cycle of referrals to the services that are known to mental health professionals and that specialize in serving psychiatric patients. While specialized services tend to be more sensitive, they also perpetuate a reliance on putting psychiatric patients out of sight and mind.

Good Intentions OverRuled

By tracing occupational therapists' experiences of tension, we can now see that such experiences are not haphazard or isolated; rather, they arise along a line of fault, a disjuncture that locates occupational therapy at the intersection of divergent methods of organization. To manage such a contradiction, occupational therapists practise with what Smith calls a 'bifurcated consciousness' (Smith, 1987). We subjectively know how the routine organization of mental health services limits practice; but daily practice is conducted with an optimism and pride that render practitioners unconscious of this organizational knowledge and the contradictions of trying to enable empowerment while perpetuating dependence, of enabling participation while preserving a system of caregiving.

The ideal outcome of including occupational therapy on a mental health 'team' or in a community is that people whom others marginalize, such as those with mental health problems, will become empowered to live productive lives. Ideally, vulnerable or disadvantaged people will develop the personal capacity and opportunity to

FIGURE 8.3
Good Intentions OverRuled

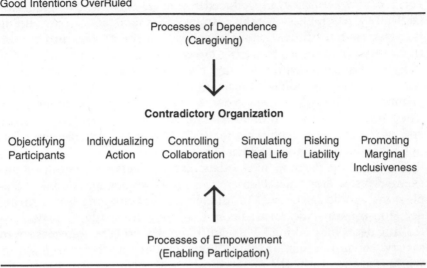

work, play, and generally share the power and resources of their communities. In the daily practice of mental health day programs, we have evidence that occupational therapists actually enable participation in ways that are consistent with empowerment, enabling people to participate, to some degree, in some occupations they find useful and meaningful in their environment. These aspects of practice demonstrate examples of ideal occupational therapy and of empowerment; unfortunately, they make occupational therapists misfits in the routine organization of mental health services.

The overwhelming evidence is that empowerment is overruled, as occupational therapists, with everyone else, comply with the routine processes of objectification, individualized accountability, hierarchical decision making, standardized and simulation-based education, risk management, and exclusion. These organizational processes, acting together and anonymously, form the dependency-producing ruling apparatus of mental health services. Empowerment processes contravene the prevailing processes of dependence, but processes of dependence diminish any real empowerment potential. The resulting practice is fraught with the contradictions displayed in the six features of occupational therapy summarized in figure 8.3.

To begin with, there is a contradiction in 'objectifying participants.' People are certainly participants, but their active potential is objectified when they are reduced to cases. Second, day programs facilitate participants to take responsibility and action in helping themselves, but occupational therapists find themselves in the contradictory position of promoting broad-ranging collective as well as individual actions, while defining and recording this action largely with reference to individual case management. Social action exists primarily as invisible, unpaid work completed on volunteer time. They find themselves 'individualizing action' because professionals and programs are accountable for individual case management, but not for collective action or social change.

Third, while participants collaborate in decision making about themselves and specific elements of programs, occupational therapists are at odds between simultaneously encouraging but limiting decision making, the result being that they are inadvertently 'controlling decision making.' This contradictory process is necessary to satisfy consumer demands for involvement in decision making, while also sustaining the hierarchical organization in which patients are dependent on the professionals, managers, and corporate executives who control what can be done in mental health services.

Fourth, day programs emphasize critical reflection and experiential learning; yet education is based on simulated experiences in standardized conditions. Despite a professional commitment to engage people in useful and meaningful occupations in their environment, occupational therapists actively limit empowerment education by engaging people in the contradictory process of 'simulating real life.' They simultaneously attend to practical issues in real life while using simulation, leaving people with little educational guidance to transfer their learning to real life.

Fifth, risk taking is supported within programs; but enabling people to take risks means that occupational therapists are 'risking liability.' Tension exists in that risk taking is simultaneously emphasized and controlled so that people are challenged to participate as long as professional and institutional liability are not greatly at risk.

Sixth, inclusiveness is strongly supported among day program participants. The disjuncture is deep here because 'promoting marginal inclusiveness' is both liberating and confining. People are encouraged to feel a sense of belonging as members of a mental health community; but this is a marginal, stigmatizing community. Social and economic exclusion from the ordinary community is preserved by a referral cycle that keeps people attached to mental health services, and by an exclusionary approach to social welfare that stigmatizes and segregates people through charitable caregiving.

In the end, instances of enabling participation, which involve people in helping them achieve their own empowerment, are dominated by the prevailing organization, which is oriented toward caregiving, not empowerment.

Future Challenges: Changing the Routine Organization of Power

If the present challenges are to uncover the disjuncture that gives rise to tension in professional practice, future challenges lie in promoting change. As we discover how mental health services work, we gain knowledge to change the routine organization of power that promotes caregiving over empowerment.

A cynical person might interpret my examples of empowerment as seductive methods that blind people to their real dependence. Or instances such as those described may be acknowledged as real but serendipitous, little more than interesting twists that present no serious challenge to the mental health service hierarchy. Empowerment may be said to be colonized in the sense that the more powerful dependency-producing processes take over and replace processes of empowerment. As well, I and other occupational therapists may be viewed as idealistic, and blind to the ideological nature of practice. An over-optimistic person may find my critique excessive. In a spirit of zeal or even resistance, instances of empowerment may be interpreted as evidence that empowerment is happening and the mental health system is working well. My optimism has remained, but my awareness of organizational constraints has convinced me that change is needed.

With the ethnographic analysis as a road map, let us consider how we could organize professional services in an institution such as mental health services. The changes suggested here require professionals and managers to make major shifts. Advocacy for change is already coming from outside mental health services by people who recognize that they can be active participants, rather than cases or patients. From my professional perspective, I am about to suggest an action strategy for professionals. Before looking more carefully at a strategy for change, it is important to emphasize that empowerment has no finite end and requires continual checking.

One key part of this strategy for change is to become what some people call *community-minded*. By this, I mean developing awareness and understanding of the complexity and diversity of people's real community lives, particularly when we know them only partially in the context of mental health services. Another important aspect of this strategy is to become *constructively oppositional*. Being constructive and oppositional at the same time sounds like an oxymoron. The point is that empowerment opposes the status quo, opposes existing ruling relations, and opposes a privileged organization of power. Those who decide to be constructively oppositional are not alone, because many people would like to change the system. What is needed are analyses, such as this one, to show where change is needed. Institutional ethnographies show the interpenetration of the everyday world and routine processes that invisibly organize power, providing us with direction for change in two arenas: everyday practice, and organization.

Everyday Practice

Since empowerment is a participatory, learning process that changes power relations, everyday practice is an important arena for producing change. Changes in daily routines, interactions, and structures are practical ways of engaging in empowerment, even if these produce only localized shifts in power. For professions that claim to be client-centred, such as occupational therapy, the call is to actually *be* client-centred in the talk, actions, and structure of everyday practice – to demonstrate and facilitate participation, social change, collaboration, reflection, experience, risk taking, and inclusiveness in the everyday arena.

To start with, we might refer to *persons, clients, residents, members*, or some other active designation rather than call people patients or cases. We can respect and invite people to participate as active agents in shaping their own lives, even when we think people are too young, old, naïve, or incompetent. People surprise us.

Professionals who work in highly individualized ways might consider becoming more involved in collective action. Much could be accomplished that would benefit individuals and communities if we worked more with families, self-help groups, planning organizations, community development agencies, governments, and corporations where there is a shared interest in promoting empowerment and equality.

If we can see people as active participants and work with them in self-help and other groups, we are on the road to partnership. The implication of forming partnerships is that programs would not be designed, implemented, and evaluated solely by professional experts. Together, professionals and those who use professional services would take time to become educated for working together. Rather than use textbook models or professionally defined protocols, programs would adopt frameworks and educational programs that operate in the places and times decided on through debate among partners.

As far as everyday practice in mental health services is concerned, not everyone wants to or is ready to participate in designing, implementing, or evaluating programs. Yet learning to structure programs could be incorporated into the assertiveness, self-esteem, and skill development areas that already comprise many mental health programs. Clubhouse programs that follow the philosophy of psychosocial rehabilitation could be more proactive and public in demonstrating how both professionals and clubhouse members can contribute their expertise based on their insiders' knowledge of the mental health system. Participants' experience would then be blended with professionals' theoretical knowledge and planning experience. If decision making includes those who represent individual, family, community, professional, and management perspectives, programs would emerge that are relevant and appropriate, and that can be evaluated from each of these perspectives.

Part of empowerment involves learning to feel more powerful and to think and act with power in real life. This means that everyday professional practice needs to be based in real-life situations, even if simulation exercises in safe places are incorporated as part of the educational program. To do this, professionals who support empowerment would advocate to work where and when help is needed, not confined to fixed service locations and daytime hours. Empowerment programs might adopt a historic view of *occupations* as a framework for understanding how people can occupy themselves in useful and meaningful ways, even if they do not fit within normative expectations for employment. Whatever framework is used, simulation exercises as well as opportunities for critical reflection and participatory learning would be designed collaboratively, by those who have experienced difficulties consulting with professionals. Collaborative planning would also help to guide the transfer of learning from simulation to real life.

What about risk taking? Professionals would enable participants to explore what is realistic given their ability and readiness to take risks. Professionals might also take some risks – giving weight to subjective experience as well as professional expertise, and sharing privileges with participants. Shared risk taking could be negotiated as a way of clarifying the responsibilities and actions that each partner is taking on. The point is not to abandon professional responsibility, but to draw people into learning to judge when they are ready to share in challenges, responsibilities, and risk taking. Contracts would be drawn up to clarify the risks, responsibilities, and consequences for all involved.

Professionals could personally reduce exclusiveness by sharing privileges, eating areas, washrooms, library materials, educational opportunities, presentations, and chores. We have been educated to create professional distance in therapeutic relationships. Distance can help professionals to keep a clear mind, to resist the burnout that goes with intense emotional work, and to clarify the purpose of professional relationships. I am suggesting that we stop using distance to justify privilege. As well, professionals can advocate from the inside for consumer membership on decision-making committees and boards of directors. Professionals would also coach people to become their own advocates in programs as well as in their own lives.

Organization

Modern organization is based almost exclusively on documents, including job descriptions, policies, statistics, texts, reports, and other documentation. The implication is that empowerment needs to be embedded in the documents that display and control what can be done. For instance, the guidelines, policies, and forms used to access mental health programs might be developed jointly by representative consumers, professionals, and managers, with criteria that include but extend beyond a psychiatric diagnosis. Schools, corporations, and community agencies, as well as health services, would develop criteria for accessing mental health services that are organized in those real contexts. The *DSM* would be a diagnostic tool for psychiatric use, but would not control participation in mental health services. An important element of access guidelines would be to define people as participants, not patients.

To shift away from the overwhelming individualization of health services, collective action would need to become a legitimate part of practice, despite the challenges that community development and other social change have presented for mental health professionals and governments. Management Information Systems (MIS) would gather and use statistics on group, community, policy, and other work as well as the work with individuals. An expanded MIS database could be used to make programs accountable for inviting participation and working in partnerships in collective and individual action. Monthly and annual reports would report not only on individual cases but also on group participation, collaboration, and community integration. Advocacy for promoting mental health in society overall would be accepted as a responsibility of mental health services, but policies on mental health would also become commonplace in education, employment, and other arenas. To reduce the potential charges of conflict of interest from community businesses and political leaders, collective action would need to be developed in partnerships involving mental health consumers as well as mental health professionals, policy analysts, and businesspeople. A clear mission and methods of accountability would be needed to make individual and collective empowerment a priority over financial advancement for an exclusive few.

Collaborative decision making is a major departure from the traditional hierarchical organization of mental health and other state services. Although hierarchy is deeply entrenched, services might redefine their efficiency in terms of time used in addressing community living outcomes. Quality management might emphasize processes of collaborative decision making to ensure that professionals are facilitating equal participation. The current trend to increase consumer participation on boards of directors and committees would be accelerated and expanded so that those who have experienced mental health problems have the same weight in decision making as professionals and managers. Evaluation is already becoming client-centred in inviting comments on consumer satisfaction. A more fundamental collaboration would be to form participatory research teams in which professionals, managers, and those using services mutually define the questions, data gathering, analysis, and presentation of evaluation and other research findings. It is these findings, not professional or managerial ideas, that would be used to guide decisions in the reform of mental health services.

Documentation, policies, and accountability might be reorganized to support the graduated risk-taking needed to achieve empowerment. The risk-taking aspect of empowerment is particularly delicate because mental health services collaborate with the state in sustaining social control. If experiential and professional knowledge are to be given equal value, risk management policies might require professionals to prompt people to participate in deciding when to take risks and when real danger is imminent. Some provinces are already experimenting with legal health directives in which people designate someone they trust to request particular treatments and refuse others. Directives can specify the conditions (length of time, circumstances, documentation needed, etc.) under which trusted people can take charge. A major thrust would be to create legislated forms of shared documentation and liability in situations of risk taking. To this end, contracts might be developed that encourage professionals to coach people through risk taking that the partnership has determined seems appropriate. Professional and lay codes of ethics could be developed to define risk, responsibility, and liability as a shared partnership. Professional licensing would need to define risk taking as a legitimate professional practice, with guidelines provided to indicate how risks will be shared and documented. Malpractice clauses in licensing and insurance would also need to make the distinction between shared risk taking and unsafe or bad practice. Consumers, with or without professional collaboration, could educate each other about ethical responsibilities through community college or other courses, just as professionals would learn how to trust consumers and others who have nonprofessional perspectives and experience.

A particularly challenging arena for reorganizing mental health services is in welfare and market practices. Professionals and others are already advocating to replace stigmatizing welfare and unemployment insurance with more reasonable employment opportunities and financial incentives. Interestingly, in 1996, Canada actually changed its *un*employment insurance into an employment insurance program, while also changing the system of benefits. I look positively on this shift even though economic and social conditions mean that equal opportunities for meaningful employment are a long way off. For mental health services, there is an extra step: that is, to reduce the cycle of referrals among professional psychiatric services. Professionals would need to be freer to advocate for nonprofessional community services to support people in living with mental health problems, even if some professional contact is sustained. There is no need for people with mental health problems to be isolated in communities, given the numbers of people and services interested in providing supportive housing, employment, and recreation. The key is to develop funding mechanisms in mental health and other services to expand services that support daily living and reduce the need for expensive, stigmatizing medical follow-up.

As well, to promote inclusiveness and change the exclusion produced by the caregiving approaches of social welfare, professionals would press institutions such as mental health services to restructure budgets and financial priorities. Where self-help groups, peer coaches, and others with experiential knowledge become involved in services, we might create fee schedules that acknowledge diverse contributions, just as salaries compensate professionals for their work. If all partners have some financial support, each could be officially expected to contribute in developing mission statements, job descriptions, workload measures, health and social records, quality assurance and audit criteria, accreditation, and management information systems.

Some provincial mental health services are already offering financial incentives to a host of housing, recreation, community action, and employment initiatives. However, consumer-run businesses, housing cooperatives, and self-help groups still have difficulty gaining the financial support of ordinary development agencies and financial institutions. Professionals, then, are called on to advocate for more federal, provincial, and municipal mental health service funding for supportive housing, transitional employment, supportive employment, and other programs. Governments, in turn, need to accept advocacy as a legitimate part of professional mental health practice and as an important approach for reducing the exclusionary effect of social welfare. A sympathetic, well-informed professional voice could join with consumers in replacing institutional residences, sheltered workshops, and special recreation with a range of guaranteed entitlements so that those with diverse needs are included in ordinary life.

In these times, we need to think about the influence that decentralized and regionalized modes of governance have on empowerment. Mental health services, like all modern institutions, are not only de-institutionalizing but also regionalizing services. Professionals who promote empowerment would rejoice in the potential for enhancing local participation in regionalized decision making. However, we also need to advocate for regional involvement in centralized decision making about funding and policies that shape the overall structure of services. Professionals who are conscious of organization and power can work with regional groups to develop management information systems, policies, budgets, and other documentation that provide regional control and central participation in decision making. In public meetings, letters to newspapers, media talks, and other nonprofessional situations, professionals could help people to embed empowerment in regionalization so that it becomes more than a rationalization of services.

As professionals, we have a responsibility to make sure that we are not losing the equalizing function of national policies in the name of efficiency. Some localized services may be enlightened, professionals are needed to band with local people to ensure that the state can create equal opportunities for those in rural and urban areas, and for everyone regardless of gender, race, or other characteristic. There is an urgent need for professionals to speak out with others against current trends to reduce the role of government in equalizing opportunities, because local compassion tends to generate food banks and other subsistence forms of caregiving, not empowerment. Professionals are needed to raise caution about the growing reliance on philanthropy from individual citizens and corporations as the state relinquishes its responsibility for legislating entitlement to share power and resources. As Navarro (1991, p. 609) argues:

The solution is to call not for compassion, but for solidarity and for universal social policies that do not preempt special emphasis on programs for those who are especially vulnerable.

If we are to make radical shifts to reorganize power, we need enlightened and committed professionals and citizens. Those already practising will need to examine their work through self-directed or formalized continuing education. As well, entry-level professional education needs to orient new professionals to a Profile of Empowerment, with awareness of the pitfalls inherent in falling into a caregiving mode, as in the Profile of Dependence. Students would learn to work as equal collaborators with a variety of partners. Debates, analytic exercises, and problem-based scenarios would be addressed with participants in services who can comment on the usefulness of professional approaches. With citizens, professionals might be involved in organizing courses on working with professionals, so that everyone would learn issues of consent and confidentiality, as well as the assertiveness and knowledge of organization needed to engage in collaborative decision making.

To enhance consciousness of the social organization of professional practice, courses might aim to promote *critical analysis*, *critical reflection*, and *professional reasoning*. Courses on social, economic, political, financial, and legal practices might be required for all professionals, and might be available for others who want to learn to be partners with professionals. Public policy and community economic development would be emphasized as a foundation for understanding mental health problems, and be particularly sensitive to gender, race, class, and other characteristics. Mental health professionals would benefit from connections with students in anthropology, community development, adult and school-based education, history, philosophy, management, sociology, political science, public administration, and law. Possibly, students would learn to research the organization of power through the type of *institutional* analysis raised by this ethnography.

Such is the magnitude of change required to organize a Profile of Empowerment in the work done by institutions such as mental health services. We need professionals who will challenge individualism, philanthropy, and hierarchy. If empowerment is to occur, we need to lobby for part-time, supportive, and other nontraditional employment. We need to challenge unions to accept and protect nontraditional workers. Essentially, we need to organize every aspect of life to shift away from hierarchy, status, and wealth to realize fairness, not only for those with mental health problems but for everyone.

Reflections on Taking a Critical Perspective

The route to empowerment for people with mental health problems seems long and tortuous. In and outside mental health services, people with mental health problems refer to themselves as psychiatric patients. Confidentiality legislation perpetuates dependence in order to protect people with mental health problems from discrimination at work, home, or in their communities. Added to these barriers are social and economic priorities that implicitly (and sometimes explicitly) leave these people on the margins.

Professionals tend to control collaborative decision making even within the personal realm of goal setting and case coordination. If one experiences mental health problems, one has very little guidance in learning to deal with real-life situations. Instead, program philosophies and funding conditions silently encourage services to stay within designated locations and daytime schedules. Unwittingly, mental health practice is organized to include psychiatric patients in psychiatric communities and place them on the margins of society. In a linguistic attempt to minimize stigmatization, we now speak about *mental health consumers*, with *mental health problems*, in *mental health programs*. Yet life for many people with long-term mental difficulties is still marginal, sustained by small disability pensions and services that depend on public welfare or private charity.

When professionals attempt to promote empowerment but go along with the system, we lose sight of the disjuncture, the contradiction in everyday practice. We are left with a sense of frustration at being misfits who are unaware of the organizational basis of our frustration. As with occupational therapists who work in a medical, individual case-managed context, professionals are left with a sense of being *different*, *deficient*, *liberated*, *powerless*, a *go-between*, in a *different mind-set*, or *confined*. The tension is not readily visible from a standpoint in everyday practice. Some compromise may be necessary as part of ongoing negotiations and debates to seek a path forward. Too much compromise, however, means that intentions are overruled, and empowerment is little more than a trivialized word.

On seeing how empowerment is overruled, we might ask why the situation persists. We know that mental health professionals tend to dominate patients and to assume they know what is best. As well, we understand that the emphasis on psychiatric medication does not fully attend to mental health problems. We also know that the medical profession and international pharmaceutical companies have vested interests in perpetuating this emphasis.

Looking at the situation from the perspective of consumers, we also know that it is difficult to be a political advocate if you are struggling to think clearly and to keep your emotions under control, let alone to get past the stigma you experience every time someone discovers you have been a 'psychiatric patient.' Certainly, it is difficult to make your voice heard in the paternalistic, hierarchical system of mental health services, because your ideas are often dismissed as naive or distorted, lacking the broader, educated perspective of professionals and corporate managers.

Maybe caregiving persists because we are only now becoming conscious of the routine organization of power. We have engaged in the everyday world with a bifurcated consciousness, meaning that we know how everyday life is organized, but we are unconscious of the ways that processes of power interpenetrate and are embedded in the everyday world. Perhaps the road map provided by this institutional analysis of power will resonate sufficiently that participants, professionals, and managers will be energized to develop empowering organizational practices.

A legitimate question is: Can *any* modern institution be organized to promote empowerment? Contradictions between the rhetoric and reality of empowerment are likely inevitable in a modern society that needs to coordinate and control complex functions, to create order out of the confusion and messiness of reality. The scale and complexity of institutions such as mental health services mean that coordination and control must be largely documentary rather than face-to-face processes.

While large-scale organization is likely here to stay, what progress can be made in organizing empowerment instead of dependence? At present, empowerment is overruled by organizing services, which support traditionally patriarchal professions such as medicine, psychology, and management. Moreover, the illustration of empowerment here is provided by occupational therapy, a profession practised largely by women. These two sentences suggest that a number of gender questions need to be raised. Is empowerment *women's work*, in contrast to the scientific work of males? Are there gender issues in developing collaborative decision making, especially since archaeological evidence of collaborative societies shows that they were matriarchal? Certainly, feminist scholars have challenged the gendered nature of psychiatric classification. What about seeking empowerment examples among predominantly female and predominantly male professions? Since empowerment is a complex process and power relation, not a measurable behaviour, should empowerment be evaluated by interpretive and critical social sciences, traditionally favoured more by women, than by the positivist methods that have arisen in the patriarchal world of empirical science?

Critical questions might also be raised about class, race, age, sexual orientation, and other characteristics, as they intersect with gender and mental health. Why do some diseases receive so much attention and fund raising, while research on mental health problems attracts much less financial support, except from the pharmaceutical industry? What funders would support research on managing risk in partnership, or in promoting social and economic inclusion in a market-driven society? How is power routinely organized in industry, corporations, unemployment insurance, workers' compensation, or disability insurance agencies? Reforms in mental health and other services might be evaluated in the form of an *empowerment impact* assessment to see how participation, collaboration, and inclusiveness have been increased.

At present, mental health services and society educate people to think and act like mental patients who individualize their difficulties and rely on professionals for help. Patients learn to be the dependent recipients of caregiving even if they are offered limited choices for participating in individual case management and the daily organization of program activities. What if people learned about their active power to collaborate in the individual and collective actions needed for sharing power more equitably in mental health services and society? What would be the curriculum, sites, methods, and structural organization of this type of education?

I will end with the optimistic comment that it seems possible, if not probable, for professionals to enable participation in empowerment by those with mental health problems. Some may view my optimism as overly idealistic and romantic. While I am committed to raising critical perspectives, I am also committed to taking an optimistic view: pessimism does not suit my character. My perception of the possibility of change is based on a belief that humans generally support fairness, and some of what we do can actually advance empowerment. The road is rocky and long, as Brosio (1990, p. 81) states:

Teaching and learning for democratic citizen empowerment will require resolute adults who are in the struggle for the duration; furthermore it must be realized that they must develop strength superior to the awesome power of capital and capitalist hegemony. This is not a job just for school kids and a few brave educators.

Good intentions are indeed overruled. Nevertheless we need to act on our good intentions so that the routine organization of power favours empowerment for us all.

Notes

1 Exploring Empowerment

1 Jill is one of seven occupational therapists whose everyday world of practice provided me with the opportunity to see how mental health services are organized, not in official terms but as routine, taken-for-granted ways of working. All names of people and places have been changed to ensure confidentiality. The names used are female to reflect the gender composition of occupational therapy.

2 Reference citations in this text will be kept to a minimum to sustain the flow needed for reading and thinking about the ideas presented. References have been inserted in the text only where ideas are singularly attributable to a specific author or authors. Otherwise, I acknowledge my indebtedness to many valuable sources through their inclusion in the Reference list.

3 Ideas on empowerment are drawn from many sources. Some authors have articulated the same general orientation to empowerment as is presented here, recognizing that there is an interplay between personal and social transformation. Notable among these authors are Brian Fay, Paulo Freire, Janice Kuyek, Stephen Lukes, and Dorothy Smith. Other authors have focused on particular features of empowerment. Key references that inform the book include: Belenky et al. (1986); Brookfield (1987a); Campbell & Manicom (1995); Carr & Kemmis (1986); de Montigny (1995); Ellsworth (1989); Habermas (1984); Kieffer (1984); Kilian (1988); MacIntyre (1984); McKnight (1989); Mezirow (1991); Pinderhughes (1990); Welton (1995); Whitmore & Kerans (1988); and Young (1990).

4 For critiques of professions, management, and the state (in general and with reference to mental illness), I relied particularly on: Braverman (1975); Cassin (1990); Coburn et al. (1987); Cohen & Scull (1983); Conrad

& Schneider (1980); Doerner (1981); Douglas (1970); Ehrenreich (1978); Foucault (1965); Frank (1992); Freidson (1986), as well as earlier works on medicine by Friedson; Giddens (1991); Gough (1979); Grace (1991); Illich et al. (1977); Ingleby (1981); Larson (1977); McNeil (1987); Moscovitch & Drover (1981); Navarro (1986); Smith & David (1975); Waitzkin (1989).

5 New critiques of living with a physical, mental, or social disability are appearing rapidly. Important questions have been raised in such references as: Bachrach (1988); Checkoway & Norsman (1986); Chesler (1972); Coalition of Provincial Organizations of the Mentally Handicapped (1986); Cook (1988); De Jong (1979); Ehrenreich & English (1979); Goffman (1961); Hollingshead & Redlich (1958); Liberman (1988); Rose & Black (1985); Rosenhan (1975); Scheff (1975); Simmons (1982); Szasz (1961); and Woodside (1991).

6 I have drawn extensively on occupational therapy literature, particular on: Clarke et al. (1991); Grady (1995); Jongbloed & Crichton (1990); Le Vesconte (1935); Litterst (1992); Low (1992); Mattingly & Hayes Fleming (1994); Reilly (1962); Rogers (1982); Tate (1974); Yerxa (1992); Yerxa, (1995); Yerxa et al. (1990).

2 Objectifying Participants

1 This general summary of mental health problems has been drawn from all sites as occupational therapists describe and document people's difficulties. The description has been supplemented from my past practice with people using mental health services, from many psychiatric texts, and from the American Psychiatric Association's *Diagnostic and Statistical Manual of Mental Disorders (DSM)*.

2 The 'Clubhouse' philosophy is prominent in programs described as *psychosocial rehabilitation*. One of its key assumptions is a person-centred recognition that people are active *members*. Some psychosocial rehabilitation programs eliminate all professional involvement in favour of member control and operation of programs. Where professionals are included, their recognition of members' power is a cornerstone of the professional–member relationship.

3 Mattingly, an anthropologist, has made a major contribution to occupational therapy. In her doctoral thesis with Dr Donald Schon of Harvard University and in subsequent studies, she analysed occupational therapy's *clinical reasoning*. She described occupational therapy as a two-bodied profession, integrating scientific reasoning based on medical knowledge

with narrative reasoning based on phenomenological knowledge about everyday living.

4 The American Psychiatric Association's *Diagnostic and Statistical Manual of Mental Disorders (DSM)* and the World Health Organization's International Classification of Diseases (ICD) are used by medicine to classify the aetiology (causes) of diseases, including neurological diseases associated with mental disorders. The *DSM* was developed to classify the organic pathology, psychopathology, and social conditions that are included in the concept of 'mental disorder.' I acknowledge the ideological character of the *DSM*, particularly in interpreting gender (Chesler, 1972; Howell & Bayes, 1981; Ingleby, 1981; Smith & David, 1975). However, its integration of psychological and social elements of life is less fragmenting and has more social analysis than other medical classifications. A feature of the *DSM* that distinguishes it from other medical classifications is its accommodation of psychological and social concepts of function in a system of multiple axes. Occupational therapists have welcomed the addition of the most recent axis, Axis V, which integrates everyday dysfunction and function in the classification of mental disorders (Canadian Association of Occupational Therapists, 1993a).

3 Individualizing Action

1 My memory of participating in the development of the occupational therapy Workload Measurement System (WMS) in the 1970s is that this 'nonpatient activities' category was inserted in response to strong representation by occupational therapists to the Department of National Health and Welfare and Statistics Canada. This WMS was developed for use by physiotherapists and occupational therapists at a time when the two professions were returning to their original separate education and practice after a 40-year period when they were combined. Occupational therapists argued that the system needed to acknowledge community involvement as well as individualized work.

2 I will use the term 'quality assurance' since it was used in the sites studied. However, the more current discourse and practice refers to 'total quality management,' or TQM. TQM is managed through an ongoing process defined as a 'quality improvement program,' or QIP. Accountability for 'quality' services is now an ongoing rather than a periodic check. This expectation of improvement puts practice accountability continually on the line and increases pressure to fulfil job expectations as written.

3 The change in name from a medical chart to a health record demonstrates

its function as a coordinating device for various health professions in addition to medicine.

4 Controlling Collaboration

1 Occupational therapists are beginning to analyse gender in this profession and the gendered difficulties faced by those people occupational therapists aim to help. Three of the seven occupational therapists in the study used gender-inclusive language or raised gender issues.
2 This is not to say that people have no access to professional texts. Virtually all programs have their own library or at least have access to a hospital library. These libraries tend to emphasize medical texts (especially in hospital-based programs) with only a few occupational therapy and other texts. Outside programs, professional texts are available in professional or university libraries in which ordinary people rarely have borrowing privileges.

5 Simulating Real Life

1 The term *critical reflection* has been chosen in keeping with the educational idea of reflective practice and learning (Kolb, 1984; Mezirow & Associates, 1990; Schon, 1983). For simplicity, critical reflection is used synonymously with *consciousness raising, insight development, reflection,* or other terms that are specific to psychological, philosophical, social, feminist, theological, and other discourses. Critical reflection is a process of developing a critique of the organization of everyday life – to see how power is invisibly organized and embedded in ways that suppress some aspects of everyday life.
2 None of the mental health day programs were initiated by occupational therapists. Yet the philosophy of this profession is based on the educational ideas of experiential learning. Education through the experience of daily occupation goes back to ancient times when Romans used pastoral retreats to restore themselves. Then, nineteenth-century asylums and workhouses in Britain, Europe, and North America began to employ occupation workers to educate people in occupations that might demonstrate their potential for living outside the confinement and segregation of asylums. The profession of occupational therapy was formalized at the turn of the twentieth century by educators, social workers, and nurses, who adapted Dewey's and other ideas about education to their vocational and rehabilitation work with injured Second World War soldiers.

Whereas early occupational work educated people in real experience, occupational work after the turn of the century became confined largely to those handcrafts that could be conducted within what was called *occupational rooms*, particularly within tuberculosis sanatoriums. Occupations were segmented into chunks of activity that could be accomplished during designated time segments in hospitals. Occupation workers no longer structured routines that shaped a real, meaningful daily or yearly existence.

From the 1920s to the 1990s, the overriding images in literature and photographs have been of occupational therapists adapting almost every kind of personal care, work, or recreation occupation to enable individual action in specially designed occupational therapy rooms. While occupational therapy began by organizing real occupations in mental asylums, the majority of reports on today's occupational therapy's mental health practice emphasize paper-and-pencil, role-play, and other simulation exercises. The purpose is usually defined with reference to self-esteem, cognitive function, emotional expression, nonverbal communication, or other psychological traits.

Approximately 80 per cent of Canadian occupational therapy takes place in the simulated situations available in health settings (Canadian Association of Occupational Therapists, 1996c). Only 20 per cent of Canadian occupational therapists work in real-life situations such as homes, schools, workplaces, and other community locations. Rather than challenging the location and scheduling of practice, occupational therapists seem to be perfecting the art of simulation. Nevertheless, occupational therapists emphasize the power of learning to be healthy through occupation – that is, real experiential learning in everyday occupations. See Reilly (1962); Cynkin (1979); Kielhofner (1983, 1985, 1995); Canadian Association of Occupational Therapists (1997).

3 The philosophy of psychosocial rehabilitation (PSR) is derived from ideas, beliefs, and values that mirror those historically held by occupational therapy. Professions other than occupational therapy – primarily nursing, psychology, psychiatry and social work – have formulated these ideas into the philosophy of psychosocial rehabilitation. Occupational therapists are strong advocates of psychosocial rehabilitation (Krupa et al., 1985).

4 Other team members have an interest in people's real lives and support budget allocations for the equipment, materials, supplies, transportation, and other costs required to engage people in real action in real community situations.

7 Promoting Marginal Inclusiveness

1 Occupational analysis and synthesis is a central process in occupational therapy. It differs from assessing an individual's occupations. This analysis investigates the inherent properties and character of an occupation: its demands on those who engage in it, and the environmental conditions that enhance or constrain engagement. Occupational analysis involves analysing the requirements and attributes of any occupation, whether simple or complex, segmented or integrated. Analysis may look at an occupational segment, such as chopping onions, or an integrated occupation, such as preparing a meal or running a household and family. Analysis attends to the physical, sensory, cognitive, emotional, spiritual and sociocultural requirements for completing an occupation. It also examines the physical, social, cultural, political, economic, legal, and other environmental features (lighting, tools, presence of other people, time, costs, policies, legal parameters, etc.) that shape an occupation.

This analysis also identifies the spiritual dimension required for engaging in an occupation (meaning, purpose, motivation, values, assumptions, attitudes, transformative potential). If the analysis reveals that an occupation requires particular knowledge, cultural attitudes, and decision-making skills, then performance of that occupation provides a medium for learning to integrate such knowledge, attitudes, and skills. On the one hand, occupational analysis dissects an occupation; on the other hand, it develops hypotheses about the developmental potential and/or the societal implications contained in the material, interactional, organizational, and other dimensions of the occupation. Occupational therapists match or 'link' assessments of individuals with analyses of occupations. The observable part of this linking is that occupational therapists recommend that people become involved in a particular occupation. Occupational therapists' informal or formal analyses of occupations underlie suggestions that people join a particular recreational program, apply for a job, meet with someone to see about a housing option, or sign up for a night class. The end result – handing someone a telephone number and a map of the bus route, or guiding them to locate information in a resource binder – appears simple, technical, and ordinary.

References

Abberley, P. (1995). Disabling ideology in health and welfare – The case of occupational therapy. *Disability and Society, 10,* 221–32.

Adamson, W.R. (1990). *Empowering disciples: Adult education in the church.* Winfield, BC: Novalis/Wood Lake Books.

American Psychiatric Association. (1987). *Diagnostic and statistical manual of mental disorders: DSM III–R.* Washington, DC: Author.

American Psychiatric Association. (1994). *Diagnostic and statistical manual of mental disorders: DSM-IV.* Washington, DC: Author.

Anthony, W., Cohen, M. & Cohen, B. (1983). Philosophy, treatment process, and principles of the psychiatric rehabilitation approach. *New Directions for Mental Health Services, 6,* 67–78.

Apple, M.W. (1986). *Teachers and texts: A political economy of class and gender relations in education.* New York: Routledge and Kegan Paul.

Bachrach, L.L. (1977). *Deinstitutionalization: A conceptual framework.* Rockville, MD: National Institute of Mental Health.

Bachrach, L.L. (1988). *Treating chronically mentally ill women.* Washington, DC: American Psychiatric Press.

Baily, R., & Brake, M. (1975). *Radical social work.* New York: Pantheon Books.

Baker, F. (1977). The interface between professionals and natural support systems. *Clinical Social Work Journal, 5,* 139–48.

Bateson, M.C. (1989). *Composing a life.* New York: Plume.

Bateson, M.C. (1994). *Peripheral visions: Learning along the way.* New York: HarperCollins.

Beard, J., Propst, R., & Malamud, T. (1982). The fountain house model of psychiatric rehabilitation. *Psychosocial Rehabilitation Journal, 5*(1), 47–53.

Belenky, M.F., Clinchy, B.M, Goldberger, N.R., & Tarule, J.M. (1986).

Women's ways of knowing: The development of self, voice and mind.
New York: Basic Books Publishers.

Benzing, P., & Strickland, R. (1983). Occupational therapy in a community based prevention program. *Occupational Therapy in Mental Health, 3,* 15–30.

Berger, P.L., & Luckmann, T. (1967). *The social construction of reality: A treatise in the sociology of knowledge.* New York: Anchor Press, Doubleday.

Berger, P.L., & Neuhaus, R.J. (1977). *To empower people: The role of mediating structures in public policy.* Washington, DC: American Enterprise Institute for Public Research Policy Research.

Bernstein, R.J. (1983). *Beyond objectivism and relativism: Science, hermeneutics and praxis.* Oxford: Blackwell.

Besancon, V., & Zipple, A.M. (1995). From day program to clubhouse: Practical strategies for supporting the transformation. *Psychosocial Rehabilitation Journal, 18,* 7–15.

Biegal, D.E., & Naparstek, A.J. (1982). *Community support systems and mental health: Practice, policy, and research.* New York: Springer Publishing Company.

Blain, J., & Townsend, E.A. (1993). Occupational therapy guidelines for client-centred practice: Impact study findings. *Canadian Journal of Occupational Therapy, 60,* 271–85.

Bloche, M.G., & Cournos, F. (1990). Mental health policy for the (1990)s: Tinkering in the interstices. *Journal of Health Politics, Policy and Law, 15,* 387–411.

Bockoven, J.S. (1971). Legacy of moral treatment – 1800's to 1900's. *American Journal of Occupational Therapy, 25,* 223–6.

Borell, L., Gustavsson, A., Sandman, P.O., & Kielhofner, G. (1994). Occupational programming in a day hospital for patients with dementia. *Occupational Therapy Journal of Research, 14,* 219–38.

Braithwaite, R.L., & Lythcott, N. (1989). Community empowerment as a strategy for health promotion for Black and other minority populations. *Journal of the American Medical Association, 261,* 282–3.

Braverman, H. (1975). *Labour and monopoly capital: The degradation of work in the 20th century.* New York: Monthly Review Press.

Breines, E.B. (1987). Pragmatism as a foundation for occupational therapy curricula. *American Journal of Occupational Therapy, 41,* 522–5.

Brook, R.H., & Appel, F.A. (1973). Quality of care assessment: Choosing a method for peer review. *New England Journal of Medicine, 288,* 1323–9.

Brookfield, S.D. (1986). *Understanding and facilitating adult learning.* San Francisco: Jossey-Bass.

Brookfield S.D. (1987a). *Developing critical thinkers*. San Francisco: Jossey-Bass.

Brookfield S.D. (1987b). *Learning Democracy: Eduard Lindeman on adult education and social change*. London: Croom Helm.

Brosio, R.A. (1990). Teaching and learning for democratic empowerment: A critical evaluation. *Educational Theory, 40*, 69–81.

Brown, L.D. (1985). People-centred development and participatory research. *Harvard Educational Review, 55*, 69–75.

Brown, K., & Gillespie, D. (1992). Recovering relationships: A feminist analysis of recovery models. *American Journal of Occupational Therapy, 46*, 1001–5.

Bucher, R., & Strauss, A. (1961). Professions in process. *American Journal of Sociology, 66*, 325–34.

Caffarella, R.S. (1994). *Planning programs for adult learners: A practical guide for educators, trainers and staff developers*. San Francisco: Jossey-Bass.

Callahan, J.C. (1984). Liberty, beneficence, and involuntary confinement. *Journal of Medicine and Philosophy, 9*, 261–93.

Campbell, D. (1980). The unit value system: If you're not interested you should be. *Canadian Journal of Occupational Therapy, 47*, 27–9.

Campbell, M.L. (1984). *Information systems and management of hospital nursing: A study in the social organization of knowledge*. Unpublished doctoral dissertation, University of Toronto.

Campbell, M.L., & Manicom, A. (1995). *Knowledge, experience, and ruling relations*. Toronto: University of Toronto Press.

Canada. (1982). *Canadian charter of rights and freedoms, Constitution Act, Part I*. Ottawa: Supply and Services Canada.

Canadian Association of Occupational Therapists. (1991). *Occupational therapy guidelines for client-centred practice*. Toronto: CAOT Publications.

Canadian Association of Occupational Therapists. (1993a). *Report of seniors health promotion project*. Toronto: CAOT Publications.

Canadian Association of Occupational Therapists. (1994a). Position statement on everyday occupations and health. *Canadian Journal of Occupational Therapy, 61*, 294–97.

Canadian Association of Occupational Therapists. (1994b). Position statement on health reform. *Canadian Journal of Occupational Therapy, 61*, 180–1.

Canadian Association of Occupational Therapists. (1996a). Membership database – 1995. *The National, 13*(4), Centrefold.

Canadian Association of Occupational Therapists. (1996b). Profile of occupational therapy practice in Canada. *Canadian Journal of Occupational Therapy, 63,* 79–113.

Canadian Association of Occupational Therapists. (1996c). *Code of ethics.* Toronto: CAOT Publications.

Canadian Association of Occupational Therapists. (1997). *Enabling occupation: An occupational therapy perspective.* Ottawa, ON: CAOT Publications.

Cancian, F.M. (1992). Feminist science: Methodologies that challenge inequality. *Gender & Society, 6,* 623–42.

Caplow, T. (1978). *The sociology of work.* Westport, CT: Greenwood Press.

Caras, S. (1994). Disabled: One more label. *Hospital and Community Psychiatry, 45,* 323–4.

Carr, W., & Kemmis, S. (1986). *Becoming critical: Education, knowledge and action research.* London: Falmer Press.

Carswell-Opzoomer, A. (1990). Muriel Driver Memorial Lecture: Occupational therapy – our time has come. *Canadian Journal of Occupational Therapy, 57,* 197–203.

Cassin, A.M. (1984). Management: A textually mediated social organization. (Unpublished)

Cassin, A.M. (1990). *The routine production of inequality: A study in the social organization of knowledge.* Unpublished doctoral dissertation, University of Toronto.

Checkoway, B., & Norsman, A. (1986). Empowering citizens with disabilities. *Community Development Journal, 21,* 270–7.

Chermak, G.D. (1990). A global perspective on disability: A review of efforts to increase access and advance social integration for disabled persons. *International Disabilities Studies, 12,* 123–7.

Chesler, M.A. (1991). Participatory action research with self-help groups: An alternative paradigm for inquiry and action. *American Journal of Community Psychology, 19,* 757–68.

Chesler, P. (1972). *Women and madness.* New York: Avon Books.

Chilton, H. (1990). Reflections on ... Managed or be managed: Where do you stand? *Canadian Journal of Occupational Therapy, 57,* 167–9.

Christiansen, C., & Baum, C. (1991). *Occupational therapy: Overcoming human performance deficits.* Thorofare, NJ: Slack.

Clark, C., Scott, E., & Krupa, T. (1993). Involving clients in program evaluation and research: A new methodology for occupational therapy. *Canadian Journal of Occupational Therapy, 60,* 192–9.

Clark, F. (1993). Occupation: Embedded in real life: Interweaving occupational science and occupational therapy. *American Journal of Occupational Therapy, 47*, 1067–78.

Clark, F.A., Parham, D., Carlson, M.E., Frank, G., Jackson, J., Pierce, D., Wolfe, R.J., & Zemke, R. (1991). Occupational science: Academic innovation in the service of occupational therapy's future. *American Journal of Occupational Therapy, 45*, 300–10.

Clifford, P.G. (1992). The myth of empowerment. *Nursing Administration Quarterly, 16*, 1–5.

Coalition of Provincial Organizations of the Mentally Handicapped (COPOH). (1986). *Defining the parameters of independent living*. Winnipeg, MN: Author.

Coburn, D. (1988). Canadian medicine: Dominance or proletarianization? *The Milbank Quarterly, 66*, 92–116.

Coburn, D. (1993). State authority, medical dominance, and trends in the regulation of the health professions: The Ontario case. *Social Science and Medicine, 37*, 129–38.

Coburn, D., D'Arcy, C., Torrence, G.M., & New, P. (1987). *Health and Canadian society: Sociological perspectives*. Markham, ON: Fitzhenry and Whiteside.

Cockerham, W.C. (1989). *Sociology of mental disorder*. (2nd ed.). Englewood Cliffs, NJ: Prentice-Hall.

Cohen, C.I. (1993). The biomedicalization of psychiatry: A critical overview. *Communtiy Mental Health Journal, 29*, 509–21.

Cohen, S., & Scull, A. (1983). *Social control and the state*. New York: St. Martin's Press.

Cohn, E.S. (1991). Clinical reasoning: Explicating complexity. *American Journal of Occupational Therapy, 45*, 969–71.

Collard, S., & Law, M. (1989). The limits of perspective transformation: A critique of Mezirow's theory. *Adult Education Quarterly, 39*, 99–107.

Condeluci, A. (1991). *Interdependence: The route to community*. Winter Park, FL: PMD Publishers Group.

Conger, J.A., & Kanungo, R.N. (1988). The empowerment process: Integrating theory and practice. *Academy of Management Review, 13*, 471–82.

Conrad, P., & Schneider, J.W. (1980). *Deviance and medicalization: From badness to sickness*. St. Louis, MO: Mosby.

Cook, J. (1988). Goffman's legacy: The elimination of the chronic mental patient's community. A review of selected literature. *Research in the Sociology of Health Care, 7*, 249–81.

Cornwall, A., & Jewkes, R. (1995). What is participatory research? *Social Science and Medicine, 41*, 1667–76.

Crompton, R. (1987). Gender, status and professionalism. *Sociology, 21*, 413–28.

Cromwell, F.S. (1977). Eleanor Clarke Slagle, the leader, the woman. *American Journal of Occupational Therapy, 31*, 645–8.

Cynkin, S. (1979). *Occupational therapy: Toward health through activities.* Boston, MA: Little, Brown and Company.

Cynkin, S., & Robinson, A.M. (1990). *Occupational therapy and activities health: Toward health through activities.* Boston: Little, Brown and Company.

Dain, N. (1989). Critics and dissenters: Reflections on 'anti-psychiatry' in the United States. *Journal of the History of the Behavioral Sciences, 25*, 3–25.

Dasler, P. (1984). Deinstitutionalizing the occupational therapist. *Occupational Therapy in Health Care, 1*, 1.

Daudi, P. (1986). *Power in the organization: The discourse of power in managerial praxis.* Oxford: Blackwell.

Davies, L. & Shragge, E. (Eds.) (1990). *Bureaucracy and community.* Montreal, PQ: Black Rose Books.

De Jong, G. (1979). Independent living: From social movement to analytic paradigm. *Archives of Physical Medicine and Rehabilitation, 60*, 435–46.

de la Boetie, E. (1975). *The politics of obedience: The discourse of voluntary servitude.* Montreal: Black Rose Books.

de Montigny, G.A.J. (1995). *Social working: An ethnography of front-line practice.* Toronto: University of Toronto Press.

Department of National Health and Welfare. (1985). *Occupational therapy workload measurement system.* Ottawa, ON: Author.

Department of National Health and Welfare. (1986). *Achieving health for all: A framework for health promotion* (39–102/1988E). Ottawa, ON: Author.

Department of National Health and Welfare. (1988). *Mental health for Canadians: Striking a balance* (H39–128/1988E). Ottawa, ON: Author.

Department of National Health and Welfare & Canadian Association of Occupational Therapists. (1983). *Guidelines for the client-centred practice of occupational therapy* (H39-33/1983E). Ottawa, ON: Author.

Department of National Health and Welfare & Canadian Association of Occupational Therapists. (1986). *Intervention guidelines for the client-centred practice of occupational therapy* (H39-100/1986E). Ottawa, ON: Author.

Department of National Health and Welfare & Canadian Association of Occupational Therapists. (1987). *Toward outcome measures in occupational therapy* (H39-114/1987E). Ottawa, ON: Author.

Derber, C. (1982). *Professionals as workers: Mental labour in advanced capitalism.* Boston: A.K. Hall and Company.

Devereaux, E.B. (1991). Community-based practice. *American Journal of Occupational Therapy, 45,* 944–6.

Dill, B.T. (1987). The dialectics of black womanhood. In S. Harding (Ed.), *Feminism and methodology* (pp. 97–108). Bloomington, IN: Indiana University Press.

Dillard, M., Andonian, L., Flores, O., Lai, L., MacRae, A., & Shakir, M. (1992). Culturally competent occupational therapy in a diversely populated mental health setting. *American Journal of Occupational Therapy, 46,* 721–6.

Dingwall, R., & Lewis, P. (1983). *Sociology of the professions: Lawyers, doctors and others.* New York: St. Martin's Press.

Doerner, K. (1981). *Madmen and the bourgeoisie: A social history of insanity and psychiatry.* Oxford: Blackwell.

Donabedian, A. (1966). Evaluating the quality of medical care. *Milbank Memorial Fund Quarterly, 44,* 166–206.

Donovan, J.L., & Blake, D.R. (1992). Patient non-compliance: Deviance or reasoned decision-making? *Social Science and Medicine, 34,* 507–13.

Dossa, P.A. (1992). Ethnography as narrative discourse: Community integration of people with developmental disabilities. *Rehabilitation Research, 15,* 1–14.

Dougherty, S.J. (1994). The generalist role in clubhouse organizations. *Psychosocial Rehabilitation Journal, 18,* 95–108.

Douglas, J.D. (1970). *Understanding everyday life: Toward the reconstruction of sociological knowledge.* Chicago: Aldine Publishing Company.

Driver, M. (1968). A philosophic view of the history of occupational therapy in Canada. *Canadian Journal of Occupational Therapy, 35,* 53–60.

Druker, P. (1993). *Post-capitalist society.* New York: Harper Business.

Dunst, C.J., & Trivette, C.M. (1989). An enablement and empowerment perspective of case management. *Topics in Early Childhood Special Education, 8,* 87–102.

Dunst, C.J., Trivette, C., Davis, M., & Cornwell, J. (1988). Enabling and empowering families of children with health impairments. *Children's Health Care, 17,* 71–81.

Dunton, W.R. (1919). *Reconstruction therapy.* Philadelphia: Saunders.

Dyck, I. (1992). Managing chronic illness: An immigrant woman's acquisition and use of health care knowledge. *American Journal of Occupational Therapy, 46,* 696–705.

Eakin, J.M. (1984). Survival of the fittest? The democratization of hospital administration in Quebec. *International Journal of Health Services, 14,* 397–412.

Ehrenreich, J. (1978). *The cultural crisis of modern medicine.* New York: Monthly Review Press.

Ehrenreich, B., & English, D. (1979). *For her own good: 150 years of the experts' advice to women.* Garden City, NY: Anchor Press.

Eisler, R. (1988). *The chalice and the blade: Our history, our future.* San Francisco: Harper and Row.

Ellek, D. (1991). Health Policy: The evolution of fairness in mental health policy. *American Journal of Occupational Therapy, 45,* 947–51.

Ellen, R.F. (1984). *Ethnographic research: A guide to general conduct.* London: Academic Press.

Ellsworth, E. (1989). Why doesn't this feel empowering? Working through the repressive myths of critical pedagogy. *Harvard Educational Review, 59,* 297–324.

Employment and Immigration Canada. (1993). *National Occupational Classification: Occupational description.* Ottawa, ON: Canada Communications Group.

England, S.L., & Evans, J. (1992). Patients'choices and perceptions after an invitation to participate in treatment decisions. *Social Science and Medicine, 34,* 1217–25.

Etzioni, A. (1964). *Modern organizations.* New Jersey: Prentice Hall.

Etzioni, A. (1969). *The semi-professions and their organization: Teachers, nurses, social workers.* New York: The Free Press.

Evans, J., & Salim, A.A. (1992). A cross-cultural test of the validity of occupational therapy assessments with patients with schizophrenia. *American Journal of Occupational Therapy, 46,* 685–95.

Evans, R.G., & Stoddart, G.L. (1990). Producing health, consuming health care. *Social Science and Medicine, 31,* 1347–63.

Fay, B. (1987). *Critical social science: Liberation and its limits.* New York: Cornell University Press.

Felton, B.J., & Shinn, M. (1981). Ideology and practice of deinstitutionalization. *Journal of Social Issues, 37,* 158–172.

Fidler, G.S., & Fidler, J.W. (1978). Doing and becoming: Purposeful action and self-actualization. *American Journal of Occupational Therapy, 32,* 305–10.

Fisher, D.B. (1994). Health care reform based on an empowerment model of recovery by people with psychiatric disabilities. *Hospital & Community Psychiatry, 45,* 913–15.

Fisher, S., & Todd, A.D. (1986). *Discourse and institutional authority: Medicine, education and law.* Norwood, NJ: Ablex Publishing.

Fleming, M.H. (1991). The therapist with the three tract mind. *American Journal of Occupational Therapy, 45,* 1007–14.

Florin, P., & Wandersman, A. (1990). An introduction to citizen participation, voluntary organizations, and community development: Insights for empowerment through research. *American Journal of Community Psychology, 18,* 41–54.

Flynn, B.C., Ray, D.W., & Rider, M.S. (1994). Empowering communities: Action research through healthy cities. *Health Education Quarterly, 21,* 395–405.

Forester, J. (1980). Listening: The social policy of everyday life (critical therapy and hermeneutics in practice). *Social Praxis, 7,* 219–32.

Foucault, M. (1965). *Madness and civilization: A history of insanity in the age of reason.* New York: Pantheon Books.

Foucault, M. (1980). *Power/knowledge: Selected interviews and other writings, 1972–1977* (C. Gordon, Ed.) (C. Gordon, L. Marshall, J. Mepham, & K. Soper, Trans.). Brighton: Harvester Press.

Frank, G. (1992). Opening feminist histories of occupational therapy. *American Journal of Occupational Therapy, 46,* 989–99.

Freidson, E. (1986). *Professional powers: A study of the institutionalization of formal knowledge.* Chicago: University of Chicago Press.

Freire, P. (1970). *Pedagogy of the oppressed: The letters to Guinea-Bissau.* New York: Continuum Books.

Freire, P. (1972). *Cultural action for freedom.* Harmondsworth: Penguin Books.

Freire, P. (1973). *Education for critical consciousness.* New York: Continuum Books.

Freire, P. (1976). *Education: The practice of freedom.* London: Writers and Readers.

Freire, P. (1985). *The politics of education: Culture, power and liberation.* (D. Macedo, Trans.) South Hadley, MA: Bergin and Garvey Publishers.

Friedland, J., & Renwick, R.M. (1993). The Issue Is – Psychosocial occupational therapy: Time to cast off the gloom and doom. *American Journal of Occupational Therapy, 47,* 467–71.

Garfinkel, H. (1967). *Studies in ethnomethodology.* Englewood Cliffs, NJ: Prentice-Hall.

Gibson, C.H. (1991). A concept analysis of empowerment. *Journal of Advanced Nursing, 16,* 354–61.

Giddens, A. (1984). *The constitution of society: Outline of the theory of structuration.* Berkeley, CA: University of California Press.

Giddens, A. (1991). *Modernity and self-identity: Self and society in the late modern age.* Stanford, CA: Stanford University Press.

Gilligan, C. (1982). *In a different voice: Psychological theory and women's development*. Cambridge, MA: Harvard University Press.

Glaser, B. (1978). *Theoretical sensitivity*. San Francisco: The Sociology Press.

Glenister, D. (1994). Patient participation in psychiatric services: A literature review and proposal for a research strategy. *Journal of Advanced Nursing, 19*, 802–11.

Goffman, E. (1961). *Asylums: Essays on the social situation of mental patients and other inmates*. New York: Anchor Press.

Gottlieb, B.H., & Coppard, A.E. (1987). Using social network therapy to create support systems for the chronically mentally disabled. *Canadian Journal of Community Mental Health, 6*, 117–31.

Gough, I. (1979). *Political economy of the welfare state*. London: MacMillan Press.

Grace, V.M. (1991). The marketing of empowerment and the construction of the health consumer: A critique of health promotion. *International Journal of Health Services, 21*, 329–43.

Grady, A.P. (1995). Building inclusive community: A challenge for occupational therapy. *American Journal of Occupational Therapy, 49*, 300–10.

Greenwood, D.J., Whyte, W.F., & Harkavy, I. (1993). Participatory action research as a process and as a goal. *Human Relations, 46*, 175–92.

Greenwood, R., Schriner, K.F., & Johnson, V. (1991). Employer concerns regarding workers with disabilities and the business-rehabilitation partnership: The PWI practitioners' perspective. *Journal of Rehabilitation, 57*, 21–5.

Gregor, F. (1994). *The social organization of knowledge in the educative work of nursing*. Unpublished doctoral dissertation, Dalhousie University, Halifax, NS.

Gruber, J., & Trickett, E.J. (1987). Can we empower others? The paradox of empowerment in the governing of an alternative public school. *American Journal of Community Psychology, 15*, 353–71.

Guba, E.G., & Lincoln, Y.S. (1989). *Fourth generation evaluation*. Newbury Park, CA: Sage Publications.

Gutting, G. (1989). *Michel Foucault's archaeology of scientific reason*. Cambridge: Cambridge University Press.

Habermas, J. (1973). *Theory and practice*. (J. Viertel, Trans.). Boston: Beacon Press.

Habermas, J. (1984). *The theory of communicative action: Volume 1. Reason and the rationalization of society*. Boston: Beacon Press.

Hall, B.L. (1981). Participatory research, popular knowledge and power: A personal reflection. *Convergence, 3*, 6–17.

Hamlin, R.B. (1992). Embracing our past, informing our future: A feminist re-vision of health care. *American Journal of Occupational Therapy, 46,* 1028–35.

Hamlin, R.B., Loukas, K.M., Froehlich, J., & MacRae, N. (1992). Feminism: An inclusive perspective. *American Journal of Occupational Therapy, 46,* 967–70.

Hammersley, M., & Atkinson, P. (1983). *Ethnography: Principles and practice.* New York: Tavistock Publications.

Harding, S. (1986). *The science question in feminism.* Ithaca, NY: Cornell University Press.

Harding, S. (1987). *Feminism and methodology.* Bloomington, IN: Open University Press.

Hawks, J.H. (1991). Power: A concept analysis. *Journal of Advanced Nursing, 16,* 754–62.

Health Canada & Canadian Association of Occupational Therapists (CAOT). (1993). *Occupational therapy guidelines for client-centred mental health practice.* Toronto: CAOT Publications.

Hearn, J. (1982). Notes on patriarchy, professionalization and the semi-professions. *Sociology, 16,* 184–202.

Holland, A. (1972). Professionalization as an historical concept. *Lock Haven Review, 13,* 52–7.

Hollingshead, A.B., & Redlich, F.C. (1958). *Social class and mental illness.* New York: John Wiley and Sons.

Hollingsworth, E.J. (1992). Falling through the cracks: Care of the chronically mentally ill in the United States, Germany, and the United Kingdom. *Journal of Health Politics, Policy and Law, 17,* 899–928.

Hopkins, H.L., & Smith, H.D. (1988). *Willard and Spackman's Occupational Therapy* (7th ed.). Philadelphia: J.P. Lippincott.

Houston, B. (1988). Gilligan and the politics of a distinctive women's morality. In L. Code, S. Mullett & C. Overall (Eds.), *Feminist perspectives: Philosophical essays on method and morals* (pp. 168–89). Toronto: University of Toronto Press.

Howell, E., & Bayes, M. (1981). *Women and mental health.* New York: Basic Books.

Howland, G.W. 1944. Occupational therapy across Canada. *Canadian Geographical Journal, 28,* 32–40.

Hughes, E.C. (1958). *Men and their work.* New York: The Free Press of Glencoe.

Ignatieff, M. (1984). *The needs of strangers: An essay on privacy, solidarity and the politics of being human.* New York: Penguin.

Illich, I. (1978). *Toward a history of needs*. New York: Pantheon Books.

Illich, I., Zola, I.K., McNight, J., Caplan, J., & Shaiken, H. (1977). *Disabling professions*. London: Marion Boyers.

Ingleby, D. (1981). *Critical psychiatry: The politics of mental health*. Middlesex: Penguin.

Irvine, S.R. (1980). Occupational therapy and the need to influence delivery of service. *Canadian Journal of Occupational Therapy, 47*, 59.

Israel, B.A., Schurman, S.J., & Hugentobler, M.K. (1992). Conducting action research: Relationships between organization members and researchers. *Journal of Applied Behavioral Science, 28*, 74–101.

Jackson, N.S. (1990). Wolves in charge of the chicken coop: Competence as good management. In J. Muller (Ed.), *Education for Work – Education as Work: Canada's Changing Community Colleges* (pp. 113–24). Toronto: Garamond.

Johnson, J.A., & Yerxa, E.J. (1989). *Occupational science: The foundation for new models of practice*. New York: Haworth.

Johnson, T.J. (1972). *The professions and power*. London: Macmillan Press.

Jongbloed, L., & Crichton, A. (1990). A new definition of disability: Implications for rehabilitation practice and social policy. *Canadian Journal of Occupational Therapy, 57*, 32–8.

Kari, N., & Michels, P. (1991). The Lazarus project: The politics of empowerment. *American Journal of Occupational Therapy, 45*, 719–25.

Katz, R. (1984). Empowerment and synergy: Expanding the community's healing resources. *Prevention in Human Services, 3*, 201–26.

Kerruish, A. (1995). Basic human values: The ethos for methodology. *Journal of Community & Applied Social Psychology, 5*, 121–43.

Kidd, J.R. (1973). *How adults learn*. New York: Association Press.

Kieffer, C. (1984). Citizen empowerment: A developmental perspective. *Prevention in Human Services, 3*, 9–36.

Kielhofner, G. (1983). *Health through occupation: Theory and practice in occupational therapy*. Philadelphia: F.A. Davis.

Kielhofner, G. (1985). The demise of diffidence: An agenda for occupational therapy. *Canadian Journal of Occupational Therapy , 52*, 165–71.

Kielhofner, G. (1992). *Conceptual foundations of occupational therapy*. Philadelphia: F.A. Davis.

Kielhofner, G. (1993). The Issue Is – Functional assessment: Toward a dialectical view of person-environment relations. *American Journal of Occupational Therapy, 47*, 248–51.

Kielhofner, G. (1995). *A model of human occupation: Theory and application, 2nd Edition*. Baltimore, MD: Williams and Wilkins.

Kilian, A. (1988). Conscientization: An empowering, nonformal education approach for community health workers. *Community Development Journal, 23*, 117–23.

Kinebanian, A., & Stomph, M. (1992). Cross-cultural occupational therapy: A critical reflection. *American Journal of Occupational Therapy, 46*, 751–7.

King, L.J. (1978). Toward a science of adaptive responses. *American Journal of Occupational Therapy, 32*, 429–37.

Kirby, S., & McKenna, K. (1989). *Experience, research, social change: Methods from the margins.* Toronto: Garamond.

Kirk, S.A., & Kutchins, H. (1992). *The selling of DSM: The rhetoric of science in psychiatry.* New York: Aldine de Gruyter.

Kittrie, N. (1971). *The right to be different: Deviance and enforced therapy.* Baltimore: Johns Hopkins University Press.

Knowles, M.S. (1975). *Self-directed learning: A guide for learners and teachers.* Chicago: Follett Publishing.

Kolb, D.A. (1984). *Experiential learning: Experience as the source of learning and development.* Englewood Cliffs, NJ: Prentice-Hall.

Korten, D. (1984). People-centred development: Toward a framework. In D. Korten and R. Klauss (Eds.), *People-centred development: Contributions toward theory and planning frameworks.* West Hartford, CT: Kumarian.

Krefting, L. (1992). Strategies for the development of occupational therapy in the third world. *American Journal of Occupational Therapy, 46*, 758–61.

Kropotkin, P. (1989). *Mutual aid: A factor of evolution.* Montreal: Black Rose Books.

Krupa, T., & Clark, C.C. (1995). Occupational therapists as case managers: Responding to current approaches to community mental health service delivery. *Canadian Journal of Occupational Therapy, 62*, 16–22.

Krupa, T., Hayashi, C., Murphy, M., & Thornton, J. (1985). Occupational therapy issues in the treatment of the long-term mentally ill. *Canadian Journal of Occupational Therapy, 52*, 107–11.

Krupa, T., Singer, B., & Goering, P. (1988). From hospital to community. *Canadian Nurse, 84*, 14–16.

Kupers, T.A. (1993). Psychotherapy, neutrality, and the role of activism. *Community Mental Health Journal, 29*, 523–33.

Kuyek, J.N. (1990). *Fighting for hope: Organizing to realize our dreams.* Montreal: Black Rose Books.

Labonte, R. (1989a). Community empowerment: The need for political analysis. *Canadian Journal of Public Health, 80*, 87–8.

Labonte, R. (1989b). Community and professional empowerment. *Canadian Nurse* (March), 23–8.

Lamb, H.R. (1994). Only good news is politically correct. *Hospital and Community Psychiatry, 45*, 517.

Lamoureux, H., Mayer, R., & Panet-Raymond, J. (1989). *Community action.* Montreal: Black Rose Books.

Larson, M.S. (1977). *The rise of professionalism: A sociological analysis.* Berkeley, CA: University of California Press.

Lasch, C. (1977). *Haven in a heartless world: The family besieged.* New York: Basic Books.

Lasch, C. (1984). *The minimal self: Psychic survival in troubled times.* New York: W.W. Norton.

Law, M. (1991). Muriel Driver Memorial Lecture: The environment: A focus for occupational therapy. *Canadian Journal of Occupational Therapy, 58*, 171–80.

Law, M., Baptiste, S., McColl, M.A., Opzoomer, A., Polatajko, H., & Pollock, N. (1990). The Canadian occupational performance measure: An outcome measure for occupational therapy. *Canadian Journal of Occupational Therapy, 57*, 82–7.

Leighton, A.H. (1982). *Caring for mentally ill people: Psychological and social barriers in historical context.* Cambridge: Cambridge University Press.

Lesemann, F. (1984). *Services and circuses: Community and the welfare state.* Montreal: Black Rose Books.

LeVesconte, H.P. (1935). Expanding fields of occupational therapy. *Canadian Journal of Occupational Therapy, 3*, 4–12.

Levine, R.E. (1987). Looking back – The influence of the Arts and Crafts Movement on the professional status of occupational therapy. *American Journal of Occupational Therapy, 41*, 248–54.

Liberman, R. (1988). Coping with chronic mental disorders: A framework for hope. In R. Liberman (Ed.), *Psychiatric rehabilitation of chronic mental patients* (pp. 1–23). Washington, DC: American Psychological Press.

Liberman, R.P. (1994). Treatment and rehabilitation of the seriously mentally ill in China: Impressions of a society in transition. *American Journal of Orthopsychiatric, 64*, 68–77.

Lincoln, Y.S. (1992). Fourth generation evaluation, the paradigm revolution and health promotion. *Canadian Journal of Public Health, 83S1*, S6–S10.

Lincoln, Y.S., & Guba, E.G. (1985). *Naturalistic Enquiry.* Newbury Park, CA: Sage Publications.

Link, B.G., Mirotznick, J., & Cullen, F.T. (1991). The effectiveness of stigma coping orientations: Can negative consequences of mental illness labeling be avoided? *Journal of Health and Social Behavior, 32,* 302–30.

Litterst, T.A.E. (1992). Occupational therapy: The role of ideology in the development of a profession for women. *American Journal of Occupational Therapy, 46,* 20–5.

Littlewood, R. (1991). Psychiatric diagnosis and racial bias: Empirical and interpretative approaches. *Social Science and Medicine, 34,* 141–9.

Llorens, L.A. (1970). Facilitating growth and development, the promise of occupational therapy. *American Journal of Occupational Therapy, 24,* 1–9.

Lord, J., & McKillop-Farlow, D. (1990). A study of personal empowerment: Implications for health promotion. *Health Promotion* (Fall), 2–8.

Low, J.F. (1992). The reconstruction aides. *American Journal of Occupational Therapy, 46,* 38–44.

Lukes, S. (1974). *Power: A radical view.* New York: MacMillan Press.

Lukes, S. (1986). *Power.* New York: New York University Press.

MacIntyre, A. (1984). *After virtue* (2nd ed.). Notre Dame, IN: University of Notre Dame Press.

Maguire, P. (1987). *Doing participatory research: A feminist approach.* Amherst, MA: Center for International Education, University of Massachusetts.

Manen, M.V. (1990). Beyond assumptions: Shifting the limits of action research. *Theory Into Practice, 29,* 152–7.

Manicom, A. (1988). *Constituting class relations: The social organization of teachers' work.* Unpublished doctoral dissertation, University of Toronto.

Marantz, P.R. (1990). Blaming the victim: The negative consequence of preventive medicine. *American Journal of Public Health, 80,* 1186–87.

Martin, J. (1991). Special Report. The mental health professional and social action. *American Journal of Orthopsychiatric, 61,* 484–8.

Marx, K., & Engles, F. (1970). *The German ideology,* Part I. New York: Random House.

Maslow, A.H. (1943). A theory of human motivation. *Psychology Review, 50,* 370–96.

Mattingly, C., & Gillette, N. (1991). Anthropology, occupational therapy, and action research. *American Journal of Occupational Therapy, 45,* 972–8.

Mattingly, C.F. (1991). What is clinical reasoning? *American Journal of Occupational Therapy, 45,* 979–86.

Mattingly, C.F., & Hayes Fleming, M.H. (1994). *Clinical reasoning: Forms of inquiry in a therapeutic practice.* Philadelphia, PA: F.A. Davis.

Maxwell, J.D., & Maxwell, M.P. (1978). *Occupational therapy: The diffident profession (Report of the Queen's University Study of Occupational Therapy)*. Kingston, ON: Queen's University Press.

Maxwell, J.D., & Maxwell, M.P. (1983). Inner fraternity and outer sorority: Social structure and the professionalization of occupational therapy. In A. Wipper, (Ed.), *The sociology of work: Papers in honour of Osward Hall*. (Carleton Library series number 129). Ottawa, ON: Carleton University Press.

McColl, M.A., Law, M., & Stewart, D. (1993). The theoretical basis of occupation: An annotated bibliography of occupational therapy theory in the 20th century in North America. Thorofare, NJ: Slack.

McComas, J., & Carswell, A. (1994). A model for action in health promotion: A community experience. *Canadian Journal of Rehabilitation, 7*, 257–65.

McKnight, J.L. (1989). Health and empowerment. *Canadian Journal of Public Health, 76* (Supplement 1), 37–8.

McLelland, D.C. (1975). *Power: The inner experience*. New York: Irvington Publishers.

McLeroy, K.R., Gottlieb, N.H., & Burdine, J.N. (1987). The business of health promotion: Ethical issues and professional responsibilities. *Health Education Quarterly, 14*, 91–109.

McNeil, M. (1987). *Gender and expertise*. London: Free Association Books.

Meyer, A. (1922). The philosophy of occupational therapy. *Archives of Occupational Therapy, 1*, 1–10.

Meyers, C. (1992). Among children and their families: Consideration of cultural influences in assessment. *American Journal of Occupational Therapy, 46*, 737–44.

Mezirow, J. (1978). Perspective transformation. *Adult Education, 27*, 100–10.

Mezirow, J. (1991). *Transformative dimensions of adult learning*. San Francisco: Jossey-Bass.

Mezirow, J., & Associates. (1990). *Fostering critical reflection in adulthood: A guide to transformative and emancipatory learning*. San Francisco: Jossey-Bass.

Miller, J.L. (1990). *Creating spaces and finding voices: Teachers collaborating for empowerment*. Albany, NY: State University of New York Press.

Mirowsky, J., & Ross, C.E. (1989). Psychiatric diagnosis as reified measurement. *Journal of Health and Social Behavior, 30*, 11–25.

Morone, J.A. (1993). The health care bureaucracy: Small changes, big consequences. *Journal of Health Politics, Policy and Law, 18*, 723–45.

Moscovitch, A., & Drover, G. (1981). *Inequality: Essays on the political economy of social welfare*. Toronto: University of Toronto Press.

Mosey, A.C. (1981). *Occupational therapy: Configuration of a profession*. New York: Raven Press.

Mulenga, D.C. (1994). Participatory research for a radical community development. *Australian Journal of Adult and Community Education, 34,* 253–61.

Navarro, V. (1976). *Medicine under capitalism.* New York: Prodist.

Navarro, V. (1978). *Class struggle, the state, and medicine: An historical and contemporary analysis of the medical sector in Great Britain.* New York: Prodist.

Navarro, V. (1986). *Crisis, health and medicine: A social critique.* New York: Tavistock Publications.

Navarro, V. (1989). Professional dominance or proletarianization?: Neither. *The Milbank Quarterly, 66,* 57–75.

Navarro, V. (1991). Production and the welfare state: The political context of reforms. *International Journal of Health Services, 21,* 585–614.

Ng, R. (1984). Immigrant women and the state: A study of the social organization of knowledge. Unpublished doctoral dissertation, University of Toronto.

Ng, R. (1988). *The politics of community services: Immigrant women, class, and state.* Toronto: Garamond.

Oberg, A. (1990). Methods and meanings in action research: The action research journal. *Theory Into Practice, 29,* 214–21.

O'Neill, M. (1992). Community participation in Quebec's health system: A strategy to curtail community empowerment? *International Journal of Health Services, 22,* 287–301.

Panitch, L. (1977). *The Canadian state: Political economy and political power.* Toronto: University of Toronto Press.

Paul, S. (1995). Culture and its influence on occupational therapy evaluation. *Canadian Journal of Occupational Therapy, 62,* 154–61.

Pederson, A., O'Neill, M., & Rootman, I. (1994). *Health promotion in Canada: Provincial, national and international perspectives.* Toronto, ON: W.B. Saunders.

Peitchinis, S.G. (1989). *Women at work: Discrimination and response.* Toronto: McClelland and Stewart.

Peloquin, S.M. (1991). Time as a commodity: Reflections and implications. *American Journal of Occupational Therapy, 45,* 147–54.

Peyrot, M. (1982). Caseload management: Choosing suitable clients in a community health clinic agency. *Social Problems, 30,* 157–67.

Pierce, D., & Frank, G. (1992). A mother's work: Two levels of feminist analysis of family-centered care. *American Journal of Occupational Therapy, 46,* 972–80.

Pinderhughes, E.B. (1983). Empowerment for our clients and ourselves. *Social Casework: The Journal of Contemporary Social Work , 64,* 331–8.

Pinderhughes, E.B. (1990). *Understanding race, ethnicity and power: The key to efficacy in clinical practice.* New York: The Free Press.

Pizzi, M. (1992). Women, HIV infection, and AIDS: Tapestries of life, death, and empowerment. *American Journal of Occupational Therapy, 46,* 1021–7.

Polatajko, H.J. (1992). Muriel Driver Memorial Lecture: Naming and framing occupational therapy: A lecture dedicated to the life of Nancy B. *Canadian Journal of Occupational Therapy, 59,* 189–200.

Polatajko, H.J. (1994). Dreams, dilemmas, and decisions for occupational therapy practice in a new millennium: A Canadian perspective. *American Journal of Occupational Therapy, 48,* 590–4.

Primeau, L.A. (1992). A woman's place: Unpaid work in the home. *American Journal of Occupational Therapy, 46,* 981–8.

Prior, L. (1991). Community versus hospital care: The crisis in psychiatric provision. *Social Science and Medicine, 32,* 483–9.

Rachlis, M., & Kushner, C. (1994). *Strong medicine: How to save Canada's health care system.* New York: HarperCollins.

Ralph, D. (1983). *Work and madness: The rise of community psychiatry.* Montreal: Black Rose Books.

Rappaport, J. (1987). Terms of empowerment/exemplars of prevention: Toward a theory for community psychology. *American Journal of Community Psychology, 15,* 121–44.

Readman, T. (1992). Recruitment of men in occupational therapy: Past, present and future. *Canadian Journal of Occupational Therapy, 59,* 73–7.

Reason, P. (1993). Sitting between appreciation and disappointment: A critique of the special edition of human relations on action research. *Human Relations, 46,* 1253–70.

Reed, K.L. (1984). *Models of practice in occupational therapy.* Baltimore, MD: Williams and Wilkins.

Reilly, M. (1962). Occupational therapy can be one of the great ideas of 20th century medicine. *American Journal of Occupational Therapy, 16,* 1–9.

Reilly, M. (1984). The Issue Is – The importance of the client versus patient issue for occupational therapy. *American Journal of Occupational Therapy, 38,* 404–6.

Riley, M.W. (1994). Changing lives and changing social structures: Common concerns of social science and public health. *American Journal of Public Health, 84,* 1214–17.

Rinas, J., & Clyne-Jackson, S. (1989). *Professional conduct and legal concerns in mental health practice.* Norwalk, CT: Appleton and Lange.

Rogers, C. (1969). *Freedom to learn: A view of what education might become.* Columbus, OH: C.E. Merrill Publishing Co.

Rogers, J.C. (1982). Order and disorder in medicine and occupational therapy. *American Journal of Occupational Therapy, 36,* 29–35.

Rose, S.M., & Black, B.L. (1985). *Advocacy and empowerment: Mental health care in the community.* Boston: Routledge and Kegan Paul.

Rosenhan, D.L. (1975). On being sane in insane places. In T.J. Scheff (Ed.), *Labelling madness* (pp. 54–74). Englewood Cliffs, NJ: Prentice-Hall.

Rothman, D.J. (1980). *Conscience and convenience: The asylum and its alternatives in progressive America.* Boston: Little, Brown.

Rothman, J. (1989). Client self-determination: Untangling the knot. *Social Service Review, 63,* 598–612.

Rousseau, C. (1993). Community empowerment: The alternative resources movement in Quebec. *Community Mental Health Journal, 29,* 535–46.

Rozovsky, L.E., & Rozovsky, F.A. (1990). *The Canadian law of consent and treatment.* Scarborough, ON: Butterworths Canada.

Rozovsky, L.E., & Rozovsky, F.A. (1992). *Canadian health information: A legal and risk management guide* (2nd ed.). Markham, ON: Butterworths Canada.

Rueschemeyer, D. (1986). *Power and the division of labour.* Cambridge: Polity.

Ryan, W. (1976). *Blaming the victim.* New York: Vintage.

Sabshin, M. (1992). Report of the medical director. *American Journal of Psychiatry, 149,* 1434–44.

Scheff, T.J. (1963). The role of the mentally ill and the dynamics of mental disorder: A research framework. *Sociometry, 26,* 436–53.

Scheff, T.J. (Ed.). (1975). *Labelling madness.* Englewood Cliffs, NJ: Prentice-Hall.

Scheid, T.L., & Anderson, C. (1995). Living with chronic mental illness: Understanding the role of work. *Community Mental Health Journal, 31,* 163–76.

Schon, D. (1983). *The reflective practitioner: How professionals think in action.* New York: Basic Books.

Schon, D. (1987). *Educating the reflective practitioner: Toward a new design for teaching and learning in the professions.* San Francisco: Jossey-Bass.

Schutz, A. (1967). *The phenomenology of the social world* (George Walsh & Frederick Lehnert, Trans.). Evanston, IL: Northwestern University Press.

Scott, S.M. (1992). Personal change through participation in social action: A case study of ten social activists. *The Canadian Journal for the Study of Adult Education, 6,* 47–64.

Sharrott, G.W., & Yerxa, E.J. (1985). The Issue Is – Promises to keep: Implications of the referent 'patient' versus 'client' for those served by occupational therapy. *American Journal of Occupational Therapy, 39,* 401–5.

Shepherd, M. (1985). *The scientific foundations of psychiatry.* New York: Cambridge University.

Sherwin, S. (1992). *No longer patient: Feminist ethics and health care.* Philadelphia, PA: Temple University Press.

Simmons, H.G. (1982). *From asylum to welfare.* Downsview, ON: National Institute for Mental Retardation.

Smith, D.E. (1975). The statistics on mental illness (What they will not tell us about women and why). In D.E. Smith and S.J. David (Eds.). *Women look at psychiatry.* (pp. 73–119). Vancouver: Press Gang Publishers.

Smith, D.E. (1987). *The everyday world as problematic: A feminist sociology.* Toronto: University of Toronto Press.

Smith, D.E. (1990a). *Texts, facts, and femininity: Exploring the relations of ruling.* New York: Routledge.

Smith, D.E. (1990b). *The conceptual practices of power: A feminist sociology of knowledge.* Toronto: University of Toronto Press.

Smith, D.E., & David, S.J. (Eds.). (1975). *Women look at psychiatry.* Vancouver: Press Gang Publishers.

Smith, G.R. (1994). Power and health care reform. *Journal of Nursing Education, 33,* 194–7.

Smith, S.E., Pyrch, T., & Lizardi, A.O. (1993). Participatory action-research for health. *World Health Forum, 14,* 319–24.

Stanley, L. (Ed.). (1990). *Feminist praxis: Research, theory and epistemology in feminist sociology.* London: Routledge.

Statistics Canada. (1979). *Canadian schedule of unit values for occupational therapy.* Ottawa: Supply and Services Canada.

Steinem, G. (1993). *A book of self-esteem: Revolution from within.* Boston: Little, Brown and Company.

Stewart, M.J. (1991). Preparation for partnership: Reform of professional education. *The Canadian Journal for the Study of Adult Education, 5,* 1–16.

Sumsion, T. (1993). Reflections on client-centred practice: The true impact. *Canadian Journal of Occupational Therapy, 60,* 6–8.

Sutcliffe, J. (1990). *Adults with learning difficulties: Education for choice and empowerment.* Leicester, UK: The National Institute of Adult Continuing Education.

Sutherland, R., & Fulton, J. (1994). *Spending smarter and spending less: Policies and partnerships for health care in Canada.* Ottawa, ON: The Health Group.

Szasz, T. (1961). *The myth of mental illness.* New York: Hoeber-Harper.

Szasz, T. (1993). Curing, coercing, and claims-making: A reply to critics. *British Journal of Psychiatry, 162,* 797–800.

Tate, S. (1974). The scope for occupational therapists in the community in the future. *Canadian Journal of Occupational Therapy, 41,* 7–9.

Tierney, W.G. (1993). *Building communities of difference: Higher education in the twenty-first century.* Toronto: Ontario Institute for Studies in Education Press.

Tough, A. (1979). *The adult's learning projects* (2nd ed.). Toronto: Ontario Institute for Studies in Education Press.

Townsend, E. (1987). Strategies for community occupational therapy program development. *Canadian Journal of Occupational Therapy, 54,* 65–70.

Townsend, E. (1988). Developing community occupational therapy services in Canada. *Canadian Journal of Occupational Therapy, 55,* 69–74.

Townsend, E. (1992). Institutional ethnography: Explicating the organization of professional health practices intending empowerment. *Canadian Journal of Public Health, 83* (Supplement 1), S58–S61.

Townsend, E. (1993). *Occupational therapy's social vision.* Muriel Driver Memorial Lecture. *Canadian Journal of Occupational Therapy, 60,* 174–84.

Townsend, E. (1994). *Enabling empowerment or managing medical cases? Occupational therapy's mental health work.* Unpublished doctoral dissertation, Dalhousie University, Halifax, NS.

Townsend, E. (1996a). Enabling empowerment: Using simulations versus real occupations. *Canadian Journal of Occupational Therapy, 63,* 113–28.

Townsend, E. (1996b). Institutional ethnography: A method for analyzing practice. *Occupational Therapy Journal of Research, 16,* 179–99.

Townsend, E.A., Brintnell, S., & Stacey, N. (1990). Developing guidelines for client-centred occupational therapy in Canada. *Canadian Journal of Occupational Therapy, 57,* 69–76.

Trider, M.F. (1972). The future of occupational therapy. *Canadian Journal of Occupational Therapy, 39,* 3–8.

Tripp, D.H. (1990). Socially critical action research. *Theory Into Practice, 29,* 158–66.

Valentine, M.B., & Capponi, P. (1989). Mental health consumer participation on boards and committees: Barriers and strategies. *Canada's Mental Health, 37,* 8–12.

Veatch, R.M. (1990). Justice in health care: The contribution of Edmund Pellegrino. *The Journal of Medicine and Philosophy, 15,* 269–87.

Wade, J.C. (1993). Institutional racism: An analysis of the mental health system. *American Journal of Orthopsychiatry, 63*, 536–44.

Waitzkin, H. (1989). A critical theory of medical discourse: Ideology, social control, and the processing of social context in medical encounters. *Journal of Health and Social Behaviour, 30*, 220–39.

Wakefield, J.C. (1992). Disorder as harmful dysfunction: A conceptual critique of DSM-III-R's definition of mental disorder. *Psychological Review, 99*, 232–47.

Walker, G. (1990). *Family violence and the women's movement: The conceptual politics of struggle.* Toronto: University of Toronto Press.

Wallerstein, N. (1992). Powerlessness, empowerment, and health: Implications for health promotion programs. *American Journal of Health Promotion, 6*, 197–205.

Welton, M. (Ed.). (1987). *Knowledge for the people: The struggle for adult learning in English-speaking Canada, 1828–1973.* Toronto: Ontario Institute for Studies in Education Press.

Welton, M. (1995). *In defense of the lifeworld: Critical perspectives on adult learning.* Albany, NY: State University of New York Press.

West, W.L. (1984). A reaffirmed philosophy and practice of occupational therapy for the (1980)'s. *American Journal of Occupational Therapy, 38*,   15–23.

West, W.L. (1992). Ten milestone issues in AOTA history. *American Journal of Occupational Therapy, 46*, 1066–74.

Wharf, B. (1979). *Community work in Canada.* Toronto: McLelland & Stewart.

White, D., & Mercier, C. (1991). Coordinating community and public-institutional mental health services: Some unintended consequences. *Social Science and Medicine, 33*, 729–39.

Whitehead, M. (1992). The concepts and principles of equity and health. *International Journal of Health Services, 22*, 429–45.

Whitmore, E., & Kerans, P. (1988). Participation, empowerment and welfare. *Canadian Review of Social Policy, 22*, 51–60.

Wilensky, H.L. (1964). The professionalization of everyone? *American Journal of Sociology, 70*, 137–58.

Wolfensberger, W. (1972). *Normalization: The principle of normalization in human services.* Toronto: National Institute of Mental Retardation.

Woodside, H. (1984). Community care for the mentally ill. *Canadian Journal of Occupational Therapy, 51*, 182–7.

Woodside, H. (1991). National perspective – The participation of mental health consumers in health care issues. *Canadian Journal of Occupational Therapy, 58*, 3–5.

World Health Organization. (1984). *Health promotion discussion document on the concept and principles.* Geneva: WHO European Office.

Whyte, W.F. (1995). Encounters with participatory action research. *Qualitative Sociology, 18*, 289–99.

Yeich, S., & Levine, R. (1992). Participatory research's contribution to a conceptualization of empowerment. *Journal of Applied Social Psychology, 22*, 1894–908.

Yerxa, E.J. (1967). *Authentic occupational therapy.* Eleanor Clarke Slagle Lecture. *American Journal of Occupational Therapy, 21*, 1–9.

Yerxa, E.J. (1979). *The philosophical base of occupational therapy: 2000 AD.* Rockville, MD: American Occupational Therapy Association.

Yerxa, E.J. (1991). Occupational therapy: An endangered species or an academic discipline in the 21st century? *American Journal of Occupational Therapy, 45*, 680–5.

Yerxa, E.J. (1992). Some implications of occupational therapy's history for its epistemology, values, and relation to medicine. *American Journal of Occupational Therapy, 46*, 79–83.

Yerxa, E.J. (1994). Dreams, dilemmas, and decisions for occupational therapy practice in a new millennium: An American perspective. *American Journal of Occupational Therapy, 48*, 586–89.

Yerxa, E.J. (1995). Nationally speaking: Who is the keeper of occupational therapy's practice and knowledge? *American Journal of Occupational Therapy, 49*, 295–9.

Yerxa, E.J., Clark, F.A., Frank, G., Jackson, J., Parham, D., Pierce, D., Stein, C., & Zemke, R. (1990). An introduction to occupational science: A foundation for occupational therapy in the 21st century. In J.A. Johnson (Ed.), *Occupational science: The foundation for new models of practice* (pp. 1–17). New York: Haworth Press.

Young, I.M. (1987). Difference and policy: Some reflections in the context of new social movements. *Cincinnati Law Review, 56*, 535–50.

Young, I.M. (1990). *Justice and the politics of difference.* Princeton, NJ: Princeton University Press.

Zacharakis-Jutz, J. (1988). Post-Freirean adult education: A question of empowerment and power. *Adult Education Quarterly, 39*, 41–7.

Zerwekh, J.V. (1995). The practice of empowerment and coercion by expert public health nurses. *Image: Journal of Nursing Scholarship, 24*, 101–5.

Zimmerman, M.A. (1990). Taking aim on empowerment research: On the distinction between individual and psychological conceptions. *American Journal of Community Psychology, 18,* 169–77.

Zimmerman, M.A., & Rappaport, J. (1988). Citizen participation, perceived control, and psychological empowerment. *American Journal of Community Psychology, 16,* 725–50.

Zola, I.K. (1975). In the name of health and illness: On some socio-political consequences of medical influence. *Sociology of Science and Medicine, 9,* 83–7.

Zola, I.K. (1984). *Disincentives to independent living: Monograph 1.* Kansas City, KA: The Research and Training Centre on Independent Living, University of Kansas.

Index